"If There's Anything I Can Do . . ."

"If There's Anything I Can Do..."

An Easy Guide to Showing You Care

by Susan McClelland

with Susan McClelland Prescott

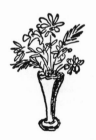

TRIAD PUBLISHING COMPANY
GAINESVILLE, FLORIDA

Library of Congress Cataloging-in-Publication Data

McClelland, Susan, 1916-
    If there's anything I can do-- ; an easy guide to showing you care
    by Susan McClelland with Susan McClelland Prescott.
       p.   cm.
    Includes index.
    ISBN 0-937404-30-6 (pbk.)
    1. Visiting the sick.   I. Prescott, Susan, 1944-   . II. Title
BJ2070.M33   1990
158' .3--dc20   90-43824
                                       CIP

Published and distributed by Triad Publishing Company
1110 NW Eighth Avenue, Gainesville, Florida 32601 - 800-525-6902
For information on bulk orders contact Special Sales Dept.

To Lee

Contents

Preface

WHY THE TWO similar names on the cover?

When my niece and namesake Susan took over part way through version 2 (or was it 3?) of this book as editor, proofreader and general vice-chairman of the project, I wanted her to be listed officially as co-author. But she felt out of place in that role. "It's your book!" she said firmly. And it is: she hasn't lived long enough to collect such experiences or such friends to teach her what to say to you. But it is her book, too. It comes to you with both our thumb-prints, both our identities.

I doubt that there are other writing relation-ships like ours. An aunt and a half-as-old niece whose names echo each other . . . that's not so strange. But what is noteworthy is that our style of writing is so similar in this book that I cannot hon-estly tell where she has entered or exited. That's quite an admission from an English teacher whom students and co-workers described as having created a "McClelland-ese" for written communication. They insisted I never needed to sign one of my notes, even if I'd typed it.

What matters most is that Susan II rescued the book, lived it, struggled to shorten, to lengthen, to clarify, to argue (sometimes diffidently) and to praise . . . in the big job of proving her belief in the book and in me. Were it not for Susan McClelland Prescott, there would be no Susan McClelland on the title page.

SUSAN MCCLELLAND

Introduction

YOU'VE JUST BEEN TOLD *that a dear friend is in the hospital. Diabetic coma. Special nurses. There's no family . . . .*

A friend calls to say she'll have to drop out of your bridge group: her husband has had a stroke and she'll be caring for him at home . . . .

Your neighbor across the street confides tearfully that they're having to sell their home. Her husband's business has failed. They're losing almost everything . . . .

Ginny, your co-worker of years and years, comes in to work one morning a pasty shade of gray. Her youngest son has had a motorcycle accident. The prognosis is poor . . . .

These are the kinds of rough going that bring out in all of us a desire to help, to pitch in and *DO* something for others in times of crisis and heart-break. Friends such as these belong to all of us if we have a home, a neighborhood, a friendly ear, a warm heart. But all too often the news of illness among friends or reports of shocks to their inner and outer worlds find us uncertain, fearful of saying or doing the wrong thing, worried about seeming intrusive or about getting in the way. Just plain at a loss as to how on earth to help.

Instead of putting our concern into action, we resort to the feeble offering, "If there's anything I can do . . . ." We mean, of course, *I want to help. I'm willing and ready. But I can't think of how.* And that's where the ball usually drops, with a thud.

But no one needs to go on like that. We may not be able to change accidents or heal the sick, but there are easy, manageable, even enjoyable ways to give a lift of spirit or a leaning place when needed. Many ways, within the reach of all of us. We simply can't afford to squander our willing and much-needed energy any longer.

And what school qualified *me* for my smart hat? No, I didn't just wake up one morning with the answers neatly laid out. That hat evolved, over a long and trying time.

What I have learned comes from years of observation and personal experience, and even more from my friends and what they did for me instead of saying you-know-what. My survival at all is tied to the efforts of those who, over the years, found ways to answer my need of help: during two long illnesses of my own as a young adult (cancer and polio); during the long, killing illness of my mother, who died younger than I am now; during the wasting illness of my sister . . . who was so close that one Christmas not long before her death she sent me the same small plaque that I had simultaneously chosen for her from a cluttered mail-order catalogue: "THE ONLY WAY I KNOW I'M ME IS YOU."

My friends lived-me-through the bone cancer that took my 20-year-old nephew, close as a son — indeed, I'd been described as wearing him around my neck as he was growing into one-year-old-hood, and I still wear him around my heart; through the series of heart attacks that destroyed my brother-in-law, dearer than most relatives who need no hyphens to define relationship; and, most recently, through the loss of Lee, the only friend doughty enough for some twenty years to share a home with me. I've had a long time to learn.

In among those gouges that tear a heart, and not always separated from them in time or place, there were non-illness crises, too. I did not drown in the actual flood waters in our basement that swirled with paralyzing speed up to my neck while outside a canoe paddled down our street. Neither did I faint in the stifling court-of-law as an unwilling witness in a custody mess and, again, in a divorce case. I have simply lived in the regular world that can move in on any person's life at any time. And, again, each time my blessed friends were there.

I've had plenty of chance to realize that, for some, "If there's anything I can do . . ." was simply something to say without needing any thought behind it. But I also heard the urgency and concern in many, many voices. I knew there was an honest, almost desperate desire to help. And it is because of those voices that I set about to write this book, in hopes of turning all that wasted good will into positive action.

The main emphasis in this book is on helping in illness because news of illness puts the most names on any list of friends we want to help. But you'll find that most of the ideas and my suggestions for expanding on those ideas can cross over into ways to hold out a hand in any hardship, whenever a reminder of another's interest and love can ease a friend's distress. This collection of ideas can, like recipes, be modified, added to, and seasoned with your own creativity.

You don't need any medical knowledge or special skills; you don't have to be a "para"-anything. All it takes, to use the ideas in this book for the benefit of your friends in trouble, is your good heart and willing energies.

I hope you're going to like what happens to you as you read. Most important, I hope you will develop a way of thinking about how you can help in bad times, so that you'll never again need to feel useless when your help matters most.

chapter one

To Phone or Not to Phone

YOU'VE JUST HEARD that a friend has been suddenly hospitalized. Your reaction is a gasp, an inner flinch. "Oh, *no!*"

Your world shifts a little from where it was just a moment ago. You're frightened, worried, filled with jagged uncertainties and shared pain. Your impulse is to reach out *right now* and pick up the phone.

It's not easy when bad news hits to think out a response to that fierce stab of concern. It's not easy to think at all! Yet the challenge of being the "right" kind of friend has to start with your first response. In most cases (and this is a bit ironic, I admit, given the title of this book), I urge you to block that first move: don't touch the telephone!

Timing

There's nothing wrong with a phone call per se; the problem is that there's absolutely no way you can control the timing. Timing is the number one key to turning good intentions into positive help, but it's also the number one culprit in turning good intentions into apparent thoughtlessness . . . or worse.

Well-timed telephone calls to a lonely invalid, for example, can be more than considerate; they can be a lifeline. A phone ringing off the hook in the home of a family just hit by an emergency, on the other hand, can be destructive tyranny. Your friend's family may already be dealing with plenty of curious others who don't care whether *their* timing is any good or not.

Here's a case in point: Last evening Betty's husband Tom suffered a heart attack. Betty has been at his side all night, and now it's nine in the morning and she's just walked in her door for a change of clothes. Thanks to the flashing red lights and siren of the ambulance last night, the word is out. Even before Betty gets to the bathroom, the telephone rings. It's Lydia Virginia, the Me-First caller. After all, nine *is* a reasonable hour in the morning, isn't it?

Meet the Callers

Lydia V., who is, in fact, little more than an acquaintance, just wants Betty to know how much she cares and how much she wants to help. She says so, several times.

That out of the way, she begins to probe for specifics. "Fairly comfortable night" is not enough. She wants information about special equipment and medication, details of Tom's activities the day before, a resume from the cardiologist. Not until she is armed with the full scoop is she satisfied that the other friends she is going to pass it all onto will recognize her for the caring person she is, and will be in awe at how well Lydia can organize her life to get things done ahead of them!

Finally free, Betty has no sooner stepped out of the shower — or, more likely, into it — than the phone rings again. This time it's Barbara, with "Lydia Virginia *just* called me and told me you said Tom was . . . ?" The question mark means: a) "was Lydia Virginia accurate?" and b) "now that you're talking to *me*, isn't there something you'd like to add?"

Poor Betty. I know Lydias and Barbaras and you do, too. They're about as helpful in a crisis as a dead battery.

The next caller is Dick, who starts off with, "I was just sitting here reading the paper and I started wondering how Tom is doing."

For beleagured Betty, this casual opener spells real trouble. It shows that Dick wants to talk and he's got all the time in the world. After all, anyone who can't simply ask, "How's Tom?" isn't going to settle for "Doing fairly well, thanks." Ten-to-one, this newspaper reader with his morning wide open isn't just a concerned friend, but a veritable authority on the illness involved.

"Gee," he will interject at the first opportunity, "I did so well after *mine*."

Depending on *your* problem, "mine" can be a coronary, a nervous breakdown, or an operation. Any reason for hospitalization that has a name also has a troop of phoners who can recite statistics, laced with advice, ad infinitum ("You tell Tom I said to cut out avocados and drop that extra ten pounds").

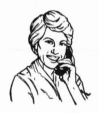

These are the same people who manage, at any gathering, to turn someone's comment about the high cost of living into a testimonial about "*MY* stopped-up sink which I managed to fix *MY*self." We all know at least a couple of these show-and-tell types. Their opinions need no urging. And while normally we manage an indulgent smile, their claim on center stage doesn't sit very well with someone who's short of sleep and raw of nerves.

Another type of self-appointed advisor who comes right to the fore in an emergency is the one who has Step Four already figured out long before Betty's got a handle on Step One.

"Now, I know you'll be needing to sell your house and find something without stairs," she informs Betty, who has been thinking more in terms of finding a fresh blouse.

"I've already talked to my realtor and he'll be glad to give you a free market evaluation. If there's anything else I can do, just give me a holler."

Betty is ready to give a holler all right!

You see what Betty's up against. I almost guarantee that she will have a whole slew of calls like these to field even before Tom is out of intensive care. If you phone now, you won't be giving Betty the solace you intended.

More Reasons Not to Call

Betty deserves prime consideration from her friends right now. Even if it's Tom who is dear to you and you barely know Betty, anything you can do to make things easier for her will be a help to both.

For she is the person managing home *and* hospital, the one running back and forth, the one who may have others at home who have to be cared for or a job elsewhere that makes its usual demands, the one who is short on sleep or food. When there's an illness in the family, she doesn't look at a clock and ask herself if this is a proper time for a nap (or a snack, or a shower).

19

Haven't you ever grabbed a nap at an odd hour, only to be awakened by a caller who, tipped off by your groggy voice, says in tones of disbelief, "Were you *ASLEEP?!*" If, guiltily, you admit that yes, you were, this somehow never takes even a knot of wind out of the caller's sails. But when *you* are the caller, you would be flattened by such an unexpected result to your good intentions.

You'd think that it should be easy enough to handle an untimely call with, "I can't talk right now. I'll call you later." But . . . no!

One part of the problem is that the very sense of heightened responsibility that keeps the person-in-charge going leads him or her to believe that the Job Description includes a *duty* to give the caller a full report. Doesn't Tom's nephew's ex-wife "deserve" to know all? I've found myself answering in minute detail questions asked by relatives who hadn't seen the patient in ten years! For lengthy inquisitions like this, even later is too soon.

The interrupted shower or bath, the endless repetition of details, the half-eaten meal that scarcely passed for hot to begin with, even the nerve-jangling rrrr-ing itself — these are strains that friends should not add to. *You* can help by eliminating that one-more call. Of course, once the patient is home, there's always the recourse for the one-in-charge to unplug. But when the hospital might call, the line has to stay open. As a friend, you'll leave it that way.

How You *Can* Help

You can write a line on a simple card to say, "My thoughts are with you. Please call me when the time is right for you." Or simply: "My love" or "My prayers . . . I'm standing by." Or any other short message that is meaningful to you.

You can go further: "Could you ask your sister to get in touch with me about the best time for me to call?," adding (if you are willing) that you would be glad to be assigned the job of phoning other friends.

Even though your note is short, you'll want it to get there quickly. True, mail does get through snow, sleet, and high humidity, but more and more it gets through on a whimsical schedule. And since you want your friend to know you do care, use your imagination to be sure of delivery.

Have the florist deliver your touching-base note with a single rose.

If you live nearby, leave it on your friend's front stoop or ask someone at the house to make sure it gets into the right hands.

The note has another distinct advantage over a phone call in that its brevity can convey real sympathy. A similarly brief phone call is hard to imagine:

"Hi. Jane and I want you to know we're thinking about you. Goodbye."

Make you feel warm and cared for? I doubt it.

21

You may not get an immediate response to your request about a good phone time or your offer to make calls. In that case, you can be glad you didn't call. Obviously any kind of phone call is not what's needed right now. You can know that your note is at least a tangible reminder of your caring and willingness. If you are taken up on your offer to make proxy calls, promise yourself ahead of time to be businesslike when you are given your instructions and to make notes on the information your calls are to include.

Wear Your Flexibility Cloak

Your friend may phone in response to your note and have nothing much to say. Have some leading questions ready so you won't fall into awkward pauses. Or, without questions, be ready to make some comments about life outside the sickroom.

Another type of friend might call and want to jabber on and on. In this case, don't get impatient, no matter how many loads of laundry are waiting. Remember, as the philospher Paul Tillich said, "The first duty of love is to listen." If it turns out that you are the one caught off-guard at a bad time, just remember that that's the gift you offered when you said, "I'm here. Call on me."

Calling the Hospital

What about contacting a hospitalized patient directly, once he or she is able to take calls? Again, it's almost always best to lead off with a note and give the patient the opportunity to do the initiating.

If you've ever been hospitalized yourself, you know that the telephone can be a downright nightmare. No matter how swank or how meager the accommodations, the single item hospital rooms have in common is a phone that is inaccessible to anyone except a Houdini. Those of us with only two arms, hands, and shoulders and a set of hips not trained to swivel are no match for the hospital-room phone, even after a resourceful nurse has safety-pinned the cord to the bed sheet.

There's a good possibility, too, that the patient has been having a long bout with pillows, pain, or the restlessness that my friend Lee aptly labeled "churchmice in my bones," and that the moment the phone rings will be the very moment he or she has finally found a comfortable position.

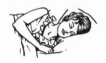

If you've ever had the fleeting thought that it might be quiet and restful to be in the hospital for a few days of peace and meals on a tray, forget it. The hospital is twenty-four hours a day of jarring interruptions: in-out, rattle-bang, a check here, a test there, roll over, sit up, and the repetition of that tired old joke, "It's time to wake up and take your sleeping pill." Finally a small oasis of quiet, and the phone rings. No fair!

23

Rather than risk adding an ill-timed phone call to the list of pills to be swallowed, why not, on your first get-well card, ask your patient to call *you*?

When You Feel You *Must* Call

There may be times when you *must* make an unscheduled call to the hospital, especially if the situation is urgent.

Let's say you're a close relative or friend from out-of-town, and there's no family to check in with. You can't sit on your hands waiting for a response to your card. In this case, you'll usually find that the floor nurse is a fine friend-at-court. Rather than disturbing a very ill loved one, ask to be connected with the floor nurse first and make a brief query: "I don't want to make things worse with a phone call. Can you tell me if he is up to talking?" If not, leave a message, along with your phone number.

Always leave your phone number, no matter how familiar it should be to the patient. Illness and medication can leave patients hazy about everyday details. Your cheerful "Oh, he knows my number!" may leave a busy nurse with a telephone directory problem she does *not* need to have.

Even the busiest floor nurse will appreciate your consideration in asking first. And yes, those nurses *are* genuinely concerned about helping their patients connect with the love and concern of the outside world.

Once the immediate crisis is past, once you have a general knowledge of the hospital situation, your own good common sense can take over. Regular calls might be just the thing to bring pleasure to your bed-bound friend.

Hospital Tips

When you know that your friend happily anticipates your conversations, a few considerations will help keep those calls satisfactory — from both ends. Stay alert to the following common sense points:

√ Mealtimes: In a hospital, these are usually very different from your idea of meal hours. Lunch at 10:45?

√ Are there special TV programs to avoid interrupting? This may sound absurd, but there's little enough to look forward to in a hospital as days and nights bump into each other, and a particular show can become a highly anticipated event. Your bookish aunt may have turned into a Cosby show fanatic. Why spoil it?

√ Is the switchboard open all night? If so, early mornings can be a very special time for a call. Patients are usually up by 5:30 or 6:00 anyway, with nothing to fill the time but waiting for breakfast.

√ Does your patient have regular medication for pain or sleep? If so, you can schedule your calls for times the patient is most likely to be alert and comfortable.

√ When you call, ask your patient if he has company. Each day may be different, and there's no point in duplicating another friend's efforts.

Plan Ahead

When you do talk to the patient, plan to carry the ball without getting stuck after "How are you?" Think ahead. Don't you have some small pieces of news not connected with the illness, like your child's latest antics? Hospital rooms are smogged with the details of illness, and your call is a chance to open a fresh-air vent.

Keep your voice calm and full of strength. If you can't be sure — if you're afraid you might cry when you hear Grampy's voice — then don't put yourself or the patient to the test. A quavering voice or sobs are a self-indulgence that's very hard on the patient, and intolerable for the person who has to put that patient back together again later. You cannot let yourself dissolve into anything less than your best self. And that's quite a big responsibility over the phone, when you can't mumble yourself out of the patient's room, or step to the window with your back to the bed if tears insist on appearing.

One of the reasons for planning your topics ahead of time is so there won't be those awkward silences or repetitions that heighten your already taut emotional state. If you fear you might break, do send your message another way. How much better than to chance a miserable call that will defeat your very purpose.

Schedule Calls

For hospital stays of more than a few days, continue your phone calls if the results have been good. As time drags on, your friend needs that outside contact more than ever.

But the gift of phoning regularly has one firm requirement: make a schedule and be obsessively rigid about keeping to it. You might think, in your busy life, that if you can't call on the customary Wednesday evening, Thursday will do just as well. But for your captive friend or relative, clinging to any schedule like a lifeboat, the missed call can loom as an outsized disappointment.

I wish I could forget some of the scenes I've witnessed — the built-up disappointment, anxious moving about the bed, wakefulness and worry — all a pitiful waste of the limited resources a patient has for the tough demands made by an illness. We on the outside can easily avoid this snafu by calling ahead of time and leaving a message if there's to be a change.

Whether or not to call? When? How often? What to say? You will decide based on the particular situation that needs your love and attention. Of course it's no Big Deal if you make a spontaneous call and your timing bombs. It won't cause real harm and you certainly won't be the only one.

But "not harming anything" is a long way from helping. In a day and age when you can pick up the phone and buy a dress, order in dinner, get the time and weather plus the latest price of corn futures, it's all too easy to dial-a-sick-person without giving much thought to what you hope to accomplish. If you just question yourself first with, *What am I calling FOR?*, then you'll be a lot more likely to start your helping campaign with the right foot forward.

chapter two

Mail Can't Fail

"SEND CARDS?" you're thinking. "Come on, now. I know enough to send a card when a friend is ill." Of course you do. But if you're like most people, it's almost a knee-jerk response. You don't think of mail as an ongoing gift in its own right, as a real answer to the question of how you can help. Yet nothing else you can do means more than sending mail to a sick person. Nothing!

Mail is the one regular, undemanding connection a patient has with the outside world. Unlike a phone call, it takes almost no effort to enjoy. It can be read once or many times. It can be counted, displayed, shared with nurses and visitors . . . even alphabetized when time drags on. Mail doesn't wilt or wear out. It doesn't require a response. And, best of all, it can be looked forward to.

Until you've been there yourself, it's almost impossible to imagine what an anticipated event the mail can be in a day measured mostly by the time between dosages and doctor's visits. Even the weakest bed-bound patient, listless about almost everything else, will perk up when someone says, "Here's your mail!" I've known patients to use mail as a reward to motivate themselves into getting over a hump. An ambulatory patient will decide to get cleaned up for the day, for example, "before the mail comes." An activity-limited patient will make the effort to dangle feet from the side of the bed — doctor's orders — one more difficult time, before opening the mail.

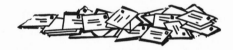

It took hospital experiences of my own to make a believer out of me. Before that, I gave about as much thought to sending cards as I did to pruning the bushes in my yard: if I tripped over some reminder of either, I'd get the job done. Otherwise, tomorrow for sure. As a patient myself, though, I found out how often I'd check my watch to guess at when the mail would come; how often I'd listen for the hall-sounds of the mail cart; how often I felt a new energy because I had cards to open.

And then I was given additional proof. At two different times in two different hospitals, I watched as a dying boy and a recovering grandmother each chose one card from a day's mail to save and open at first light the next morning. Their separate pacts with the "next" day had a lasting influence on me.

As a reformed member of the hedge-clipping variety of card sender, I can promise that for either short, hopeful confinements or for long, hopeless ones, the gift that pays the highest dividends (and for the least effort and expense) is mail.

Yet mail as a continuing gift is too often neglected. There seems to be an almost uniform rule-of-thumb with illness: send a card during the first few days; send another card the next week or so; after that (when support is most needed) most people forget cards altogether.

I think we need to change that. The longer your patient is down and the more severe the situation, the more he or she can use the kind of medicine that comes in an envelope. The effort doesn't need to be a major production, and the results don't have to be literary masterpieces. But continuity does need special attention: keep the mail coming.

Start now, one lick at a time.

Card Strategy

You've already sent that first thinking-of-you note. (Congratulations. You curbed the urge to dial!) Now you can slow down and begin to plan ahead.

If you're not one of the organized few who have an entire shelf of cards for all occasions on the ready, with envelopes pre-stamped, you'll have to do a certain amount of preparation. But there's no rush. The patient will probably be digging out from under an initial onslaught of cards for a few days.

Sit down with your appointment book or your kitchen calendar and write in Joe's or Marybeth's name at various places in the blocks of time ahead. Every three or four days or once a week— it's up to you. There's no such thing as overkill. You'll never hear a patient say, "Oh, no! Another card from Anne. How dull. When will she ever stop?"

If you haven't done any card shopping for a while, be prepared for a bewildering array. With enough hours to spend, comfortable shoes, and boundless admiration for corny jokes, you could go through card after card after card in search for the perfect *bon mot* for your cousin Marge, but that's not necessary. Don't drive yourself to distraction making selections. The "packaging" is the least important part of your mail program.

Almost any of the choices in the "thinking of you" racks are fine, with a few words of your own added before your name. Something as short as *I do mean it!* or *It's true!* before your signature can make the bought card come alive. A picture card that's blank inside can serve you very well with the addition of an enclosure (suggestions start on page 37) or a one-liner (see "What to Write," next).

There may be fortunate instances when you have time to write a long, newsy note. This is a wonderful gift, a real bonus for a shut-in patient. Don't let me hurry you! But most of the time, for most of us, there is need to beware of what I call the "note trap." Let's say your last note was a long one, so you think you had better write more this time too . . . and the next time . . . and the next. And finally you find yourself skipping calendar note dates because it's become an enormous, time-consuming production. Making your notes short and simple will keep you on the track. A brief message is enough to bring a smile to your patient's day.

What to Write

O.K., you agree: personalizing your cards with a brief message is a great addition. But for a lot of us, the thought of delivering a snappy, creative phrase on cue brings on a major case of the uh . . . uh . . . uh . . . paralysis. How many times have you stared at one of those little blank cards at the florist's (or over a wittily autographed cast thrust forward by a wounded friend) wanting to write Something, and coming up with . . . Nothing.

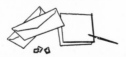

Maybe that doesn't happen to you; maybe your mind flows with originality on command. But if not, the sample one-liners and quotations that follow may help spark your own ideas, or they may work just as they are.

The sentences are not in any order, not in any category, and not for any specific age, gender or degree of illness. The idea is that *anything* (well, almost anything) that brings your friend to mind is fine subject matter for a brief, loving message.

My pen won't write more than . . . Love.

*There is no joy in / on _____
(your town / street).*

*The dog next door sure misses you . . .
yelling at him.*

Your coffee cup is getting dusty . . .

Hold tight my hand.

*I've a new plan for the garden these days:
tall weeds, mixed!*

"Laughter is an act of protest." (Auden)

*You might have opted for a Florida vacation
instead!*

*How can the weather be so beautiful
with you in THERE?*

Miss seeing your red cap (any "trademark")
when I'm jogging these days.

Can you recommend a good plumber? Every-
thing is "stopped-up" at work without you.

Super Bowl? Drooper-bowl with you away.

The Dow is up. The grass is up. My gas bill is
up. But me, I'm DOWN till you get back.

Hope I'm doing right by W. Shakespeare:
"But if the while I think on thee, dear friend
All losses are restored and sorrows end."
And I do "Think on thee." Bet on it!

The lilacs are out—OH, so beautiful!

Wish you could hear me thinking about you,
so you'd never feel alone.

The ducks are back on the lake. The leaves
are back on the trees. Now all that's missing
is you, back on your feet.

"Be still and know that I am God."
(Luke 24:10)

Every day, in every way . . . you're in my heart.

"Traviata" is on PBS Thursday at 8.
Tune in, with me?

*Our doubles match had no bounce
without you!*

No new way to say it: I plain old miss you.

*"We are not interested in the possibilities
of defeat." (Queen Victoria)*

*Webster says it best: LOVE—a whole page
of it. (Include a photocopy of the page.)*

*Browning won't mind if I borrow: "You're
my friend/ What a thing friendship is,
world without end . . . ."*

What *do* you say when you know the situation is bleak?

Just remember that the purpose of the card is *only* to make a warm connection with your friend or relative, not to shed light on how one meets death, or how one maintains dignity, or how one faces a new day of pain and hopelessness. My best advice from observation of very ill patients is to keep your message simple and manageable.

My love . . .

Night or day, my thoughts are with you . . .

These are not a strain on sender or patient, yet they do create a sometimes magic link. The cards you use don't even have to be store-bought. No, I don't have in mind whipping out the children's construction paper and blunt-nosed scissors to create dazzling effects — not unless you want to. But with a taped-on enclosure and a personal one-line note, even a plain index card is up to the job. A very small dose of creativity can spare both your billfold and your shopping time. You can also use postcards; they cost a quarter as much as glossy greeting cards and give you just as much room to write.

Once you get an inventory of cards onto your desk, you'll give yourself a big incentive if you get the mechanics of mailing out of the way. While you're on hold with the dentist's office or not watching TV commercials you can get the addressing and stamping done.

Then start your hunt for items to enclose when you choose to use them. My list or yours.

Enclosures

A friend of mine with great "card sense" once tucked a four-leaf clover she'd saved into a card for me with no comment, simply her name. A wonderful message.

A former student, remembering that I'm a word buff, sent me Word Jumbles from an out-of-town newspaper with each card.

Such simple additions bring a whole new element of special attention to a get-well message. And there are, without any shopping, endless variations.

Following is a list of good raw material, depending on your friend's interests:

A newspaper editorial.

An Erma Bombeck column.

A cartoon.

A movie or theatre review.

A bridge column.

A horoscope.

A snapshot.

A drawing by your six year old.

A pressed flower.

A short poem copied in your handwriting.

For a child:

A silly joke or a riddle with the answer sent separately.

A message written in big letters and cut up to make a simple jigsaw-type puzzle.

Is your friend an avid cook?

How about a fresh herb sprig with a note, "Can you name this herb?"

Or a recipe.

For the contest lover:

> *A sweepstakes entry blank.*

> *Or a current lottery ticket.*

For the avid reader:

> *A checklist of books you own that your friend*
> *might like to borrow. (See "R.S.V.P.,"*
> *coming up.)*

If you hit upon an enclosure that brings a delighted response, you're in luck. You may be able to use the same idea over and over: a new bridge column each week, for example. Then it becomes a kind of trademark, a treat associated with *you* — your own answer to the question of what you can do. By including enclosures like these in your planning from the beginning and keeping an eye open as you go about your daily rounds, you'll soon find you have a good stockpile.

Don't think every enclosure needs to be written words. There are beautiful pictures in almost all magazines. You don't have to make the flying gull fit in with some comment, either. As Ralph Waldo Emerson said, "Beauty is its own excuse for being." It doesn't matter if you're no word merchant. The important thing is to connect with your patient on a personal level.

Appropriateness

Call it tact, or call it good taste — it's one area where the maxim about "something always being better than nothing" doesn't hold true.

If you know the prognosis for your patient is very bad, for example, you obviously wouldn't choose a card that chuckles through a message about Getting-Outa-That-Bed or about how some folks use *any* excuse to get room service. You should also be thoughtful enough to avoid "Get Well Soon" or "Best Wishes for a Speedy Recovery" when that's clearly not going to be the case. Be careful to take time to consider whether a particular message might be a mistake.

You think I'm exaggerating? I had a dear friend in the hospital who received a "cute" card that asked, "Lose Something?" It might have been funny if she had merely had her tonsils removed. But my friend had gone through radical surgery and the joke was grotesque. If you have any doubt whatsoever as to the patient's condition and prognosis, it's better to steer clear of making light of the situation.

There's another type of message that may give rise to doubts about appropriateness. Religious cards, especially the prepackaged verse that comes fancily typeset and glossily packaged, may strike an off-note when sent to someone who does not share your beliefs. In my experience as a recipient, a religious card with an added line saying, *This verse means much to me* or *These words express my feelings so beautifully* shows that the expression of faith is a heartfelt sharing, rather than an unsolicited sermon.

R.S.V.P.

Let's talk about those occasions when you're using the mail to ask your friend if there might be something specific you can do.

Let's say you don't know Harrison very well. He was a co-worker in your office before he retired and you were fond of him, but you haven't seen him in a couple of years. You've heard that he had a heart attack, and you'd like very much to do something special for him.

You cast about . . . Aha! What about dropping by with a batch of those famous cookies of yours he always wolfed down. First, though, you need to know 1) if Harrison feels up to a visit-in-person from you, an acquaintance rather than a close friend, and 2) if the cookie idea would fly (no sense in wasting your valuable time and butter if H. is on a cookie-free diet).

So you send a card with your query: *May I come by with some of my Peanut Butter Bombs?*

So far, so good.

When you need a reply, though, a few simple additional steps can make the difference in whether or not your effort pays off for both you and Harrison. Add your phone number *and* enclose a stamped, self-addressed card, so Harrison or a family member has a choice in answering by phone or mail. Incidentally, get your last name down somewhere, whether the person is a mere acquaintance or your best friend. You already know about the very typical patient disorientation you can run into. You should be explicit enough that no one will confound himself with "Jean who?" or "What's a Peanut Butter Bomb?"

If, on the reverse side of that self-addressed card, you spell out the choices so they can just be checked off or circled, you'll have made the proposition so simple and complete that even if Harrison is alone, weak and uncomfortable, he can follow through. Maybe a bomb of a cookie would make his day, but chances are you'll never find out if you take the route most people do: *Let me know if you'd like some cookies. Fondly, Jean.* If Harrison has to figure out who Jean is, where she is, and how he can reach her, he'll probably roll over and try to get some sleep instead.

I hope I've persuaded you that mail is no trivial pursuit, an occasional addition to a "real" gift, but rather, a way to give concrete help to your friends who'll remember your great "series" for as long as time allows.

But if you still have doubts about the gift of a regular mail campaign, ask anyone who's been hospitalized or confined at home. You'll be convinced.

I'll bet my last postage stamp on it.

chapter three

Gifts to Wrap

EVER SINCE "We Three Kings," the offering of gifts
has been a favorite way of honoring friends and relatives. It's a lovely custom, surrounded by its own
special aura of generosity and thoughtfulness.

We like to give, and never more than in times
of need. Almost everyone can point to an instance
when some wonderfully-chosen gift brought a glow
of pleasure on a "down" day. We'd like to put that
kind of light into a friend's sickroom.

That's why one of the first things that comes
to mind when we think "What can I *do*?" is "What
can I *give*?"

The associations that we carry with us from childhood when we got special presents on *my* birthday, Christmas, Hanukah, or Easter are still so strong that even a knock-down illness can't wipe away the feel of a smile at the sight of a box with a bow on it.

Flowers

I can't think of a single patient I've ever known who didn't love getting flowers. Their message of hope and new life is in a language that crosses all lines of gender, age, and personal preference. Flowers deserve their rank as the first-place gift for difficult as well as for joyous times.

But do stop and think a moment before dialing your florist the moment you get news of illness or accident. (Timing. Here it is again!) The patient newly out of major surgery may be overwhelmed by an ongoing parade of cheerful gray ladies or pink ladies or candy stripers coming into the room with a florist's delivery.

You can be excused for thinking, "What a lovely way to be overwhelmed!," because *you're* not groggy or in pain. But sometimes the only way a patient trying to adjust to a frightening new set of circumstances can hang on to self-control at all is to shift into neutral and stay there. Feeling the need to come up with a smile and a pleased response every time a dozen mums are brought in may put added strain on the struggling person who has not yet had time to give over to being a patient.

Just as with cards, there's no rush once you've made your first contact. If your friend is in the hospital, the best time for your flowers may be down the road a ways. There will come a day when everyone else's cut flowers wilt, the plants look listless, and the patient is bored, hospital weary, and fighting off the post-flurry letdown. Your flowers, arriving then, bring a fresh lift.

Even though you'll be the delivery person, you don't need to tie in this gift — or any other — with a visit if you don't want to. Find the volunteers who bless most hospitals with hours and miles of their services, and ask for a helping hand in delivery. Then you can dash back to your double-parked car with confidence that your yard bouquet, in its non-valuable container, will get where you want it to go. (Now you know why you've saved all those florists' vases on that shelf in your basement.)

Another welcome time to send flowers is as a coming-home gift on the day the patient checks out of the hospital. And don't forget the possibilities of flowers in the long weeks and months ahead. A woman I know who lost her young son to leukemia receives a simple bouquet of cut flowers on the anniversary of his death. Every year. From a friend whose gesture says, without needing words, "I remember, and I'm thinking of you with special love today."

Florists don't have a monopoly on flowers. Give your back yard a chance, too, or the woods where you take walks. Your own arrangement of fall leaves, pussy willows, or spring daffodils can bring just as much pleasure as a budget-wrenching florist's version. Just be sure to add enough water for possible delays, but not enough to make a mess in your car.

Good Gifts

When you want to go beyond flowers, what then? Maybe you're after something different, unique and personal, maybe useful or entertaining. Yet you're probably not made of money and you're certainly not made of time.

In the suggestions that follow, I'll stick with gifts that are relatively inexpensive and easy to find. If they sound "dinky" to you, or if you *are* made of time and money, do go ahead and buy your friend a VCR. I won't try to stop you, but I will say that from my observation, the most successful gifts for bedridden patients are ... well ... dinky! Maybe that's because a very ill person tends to appreciate the smaller things of life and be better able to manage them. Or, perhaps, when the view has narrowed to the four blank walls of a hospital or sickroom, simple gifts make an outsized impression.

For any gift, particularly in the hospital, consider size first. Hospital rooms are cramped and quick to clutter, so pass up the giant panda bear.

A hanging crystal prism is pleasant to watch as the sun's rays hit it, and it uses no space that anything else needs to use. The same goes for a small mobile or a delicately suspended piece of stained glass. (No need for heavy hardware; these are light enough to hang with a pushpin or even tape.)

Many larger florists and nurseries sell decorative items that can hang in front of a window or sit on the sill, but you'd better check to see if there is a sill, if you're planning a gift to sit on it. Some hospitals have slanted their window sills in recent construction. Probably has to do with air flow dynamics, but what a dirty trick for gift-givers!

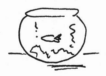

For children, posters are great. Another good idea for a child-patient is a glass-enclosed ant colony, which can provide hours of enjoyable watching. A goldfish bowl might be a good substitute if you don't have ants at your fingertips. But since the goldfish bowl has to be kept clean and the fish fed, you should clear with the parents on this one.

The big advantage of these purely-for-observing gifts is that they shift attention away from dreary medical paraphernalia. For this reason, they make good adult gifts, too. Sometimes it's nice to contemplate something other than an IV tube — or oneself!

Gifts that take mental effort and participation from the patient are worth considering, but here's a warning: steer clear of anything that might overtax limited resources, particularly hobby-type gifts requiring fine motor skills, patience, energy, control. While the idea of giving a patient something to do in the long hours of inactivity is a good one in theory, in practice it can backfire.

I once made the mistake of taking a book of Master Stumpers to a friend with competiton-level crossword skills, when he was hospitalized after surgery.

"Oh, boy," I thought proudly. "Will this ever make his day. Probably they'll have to pry the pencil out of his hand to get him to eat."

Instead, my poor friend started in obligingly as I watched with anticipation of his glee. But he was nowhere near up to his usual speed and put the book aside in frustration. "I'll have to get to that tomorrow," he said forlornly.

I've learned the lesson that the more familiar and beloved the hobby, the more disappointing it can be for the patient to find himself unable to call up his usual skills. So, before giving puzzles and games, be sure that your friend is very alert, energetic, and up to the physical and mental demands of your gift. And as a matter of practicality, whenever you give puzzle books, choose the spiral notebook form. They stay flat on a lap or a lap-board.

The same objective of helping to soak up the endless flow of hours can be achieved through a gift of audio tapes. Books on tape are available in enormous variety at bigger bookstores, or, even better, can be checked out of public libraries. Your gift could be to bring the patient a different book to listen to each week.

If the patient doesn't have a cassette player with headphones, one can be purchased (perhaps as a group gift) for a surprisingly small amount . . . or maybe borrowed. Even when the listener can barely concentrate, the sound of a fine voice reading can be highly soothing. Add music tapes for variety.

If you are long on patience—or own an eight year old who understands about "rewind," "record," and "erase" buttons, you could even make a tape of family and friends delivering messages and anecdotes to the patient. It won't be soothing, but what a winner!

Light Reading

When it comes to reading material, watch out for the hardcover book! Hard covers are just what they say they are, and no one wants to send a friend back in to have her abdominal sutures redone.

Oh, it wouldn't go that far, but a heavy book on a tender abdomen doesn't keep a patient propped up for reading very long. And heavy volumes are hard on weak hands. The big fat saga you bought in hardcover (so your friend would know you wanted him to have the very best) isn't going to be read in the hospital anyway.

Better to give lightweight paperbacks (light in both senses of the word) or topical, picture-filled magazines with short stories and human interest reading. Take a chance with that romance novel you enjoyed even if it normally wouldn't be on your patient's reading list. Try an assortment of several magazines with material off the patient's beaten track, or a collection of "Far Side" cartoons, or a Hollywood kiss-and-tell — anything that's upbeat and takes well to interruptions.

People enjoy reading things when they're ill that they'd never look at other times. I think it must be for the same reason that I'll read a children's book in the dentist's office or "The Discus Thrower's Weekly" on an airplane. I feel so out-of-context anyway that strange reading seems appealing. I know an elderly woman who spent hours in the hospital poring over *The Guiness Book of World Records*. Another confessed to a startling yen for movie magazines.

Another reading strategy that was a pleasure for one patient — so much so that she remembers it in detail some twenty years later — was a set of packets given to her with specific times, such as "Monday morning" or "Tuesday before breakfast," written on the outside. Inside each packet were articles, clippings, and cartoons chosen by a group of her friends. She didn't have to find a place to keep them because they were to be looked at and thrown away. That clever idea gave her the enjoyment of looking forward to new and unpredictable entertainment each day. She still says this was the only thing that got her through the torment of gray food and cold coffee.

My Favorite Gift

My own all-time favorite gift came with a "card" that was almost as inspired as the gift itself. A number of friends from work had gotten together to compile a booklet out of a small blank spiral notebook. The first page said,

We wanted to get you the perfect gift. We thought of a . . .

And the next page had a picture of something silly, like a tractor, cut out of a magazine. Underneath, it continued,

But we know you don't have a hayfield. So then we thought of a . . .

And the next page showed a very extreme Easter bonnet,

But it's only September.

So on and on, page after page.

I must have laughed through it a hundred times. And I'll bet it cost them no more than a nickel, an hour, and aching ribs from their own laughter.

The gift itself? My all-time favorite one? The gift I have duplicated many times since for other patients, with rave reviews?

A baby-sized down pillow!

These pillows are perfect for snuggling under a cheek hot with fever, an aching shoulder, a tired hip, a throbbing knee, or under an elbow as a prop for reading in bed. A seamstress member of the group had stitched up some colorful cotton flannel pillowcases to add a splash of gaity to the avocado-drab hospital room and to keep the laundering simple. (The pillowcases are an essential part of the gift, since they'll have to be changed almost daily with such constant use.)

A word of caution for your lucky patient who receives a down pillow: they're easily lost and *not* easily replaced. Hurried bed-changing crews may sweep the valued pillow into the laundry pile, never to be seen again. One friend's counter ploy was to simply "attach" herself to the little treasure, taking it with her to x-ray, to physical therapy, even to the bathroom. Her argument was a tough stance: "They tell you not to leave your purse, jewelry, cash- for-newspapers around. Well, they should include these fabulous little pillows! You bet they can be stolen... but not from me!"

I don't blame you for thinking I'm doing a good deal of selling for a simple baby pillow. You'll know why if you get your own head on one. Once you do, you'll find room for it in your overnight bag, your limited luggage en route to Rome, and in any bed you ever occupy. Be sure, for yourself or for gifts, that you insist on down, not the rubberized rock that's usually sold for baby pillows.

And if you can, get pillowcases that fold over like an envelope rather than the open-ended kind. The open-ended versions are too likely to let the pillow escape, especially when a patient is jockeying for a comfortable position. If you do choose this gift, you'll know forever after what you want to give a dear friend who needs your comfort.

Wearing-in-Bed Gifts

On the subject of comfort, the gift that comes most easily to many minds is a bed jacket, a lacy nightgown, or a pretty robe. But before you automatically settle on one of these regulars of sickroom gift-giving, consider that your friend may already have two or three bed jackets, probably still in their boxes. (Do you know anyone who actually wears bed jackets at home?)

Gowns are such a matter of personal preference that you might almost as easily choose a pair of prescription glasses for your friend. Besides, synthetic fabrics, frills, waistbands, long sleeves, and even buttons can be hard on sensitive skin, and patients who are handled constantly may prefer a hospital gown and a familiar old sweater from home to a lacy gown that costs far too much for such a gamble. If you really want to give a gown, your best choice may be a cotton flannel version of hospital couture: calf length, loose sleeves, closure up the back. They're not easy to find in fancy shops, but they are very easy to stitch up if you have a sewing machine.

A more satisfying and useful gift is . . . socks. Yes, socks! Plain cotton or soft acrylic socks, with *no* elastic and all one color for easy pairing, are more useful than bed socks or slippers. For a shaky patient especially, slippers can be harder to contend with than high heels for a thirteen year old. Even if a patient heading for the bathroom is lucky enough to find both slippers where last stationed, the challenge of a) getting them positioned underneath the feet, and b) "slipping" them on (a misnomer for "muscled" on, probably why they're called "mules") can defeat the whole undertaking.

Socks, though, can stay on in bed as well as out of bed (if the floors are not slippery). They are easily kept clean by the same person who might want to throttle you for your gift of "HAND WASH ONLY, PRESS

WITH COOL IRON" lingerie. Because they can be worn comfortably in bed, socks are the easiest remedy for the poor circulation that gives many patients chilly feet, and they're comfortable even on swollen, tender feet. Give a luxurious supply of five or six pairs so that there are always clean ones ready, with time for home washing and return.

I'll admit that a pile of socks doesn't look very gift-ish lying there in a box, but don't let that stop you. You can make the package entertaining, or embroider initials on the socks, or tuck in a sachet. Trust me. Socks are the one thing no hospital patient should do without.

Beautifying Ideas

If it's a safe bet that your hospitalized patient is getting a barrage of cards, think of giving a stick-up bulletin board, an album for their display, or a small basket flagged cheerily with a sign saying CARDS. A roommate of mine once brought me clothespins and a short length of clothesline, which she strung wall-to-pipe for hanging my array of cards. It was, of course, hung out of the way so as not to garrote a fast moving nurse.

Even if your patient is so ill as to be almost unaware of day and night, he or she needs to be encouraged by color, light, life, signs of the outside world. The warmer and friendlier you can help make that little cube of a room look, the less locked in your friend will feel.

If there is another patient in the room or if your friend is in a six-bed ward, you'll need to get some reaction to your decorating ideas before you go very far. But I've invariably found that space-sharing patients are happy with the improvement.

Balloons can cheer up a drab room if your patient is not too ill to enjoy them, but get the Mylar kind that last a long time. Ordinary balloons are not much fun when they start to wither.

Ask the doctor or floor nurse if your patient is strong enough for a visit (your treat) from a hairdresser, a manicurist, or a masseuse. If you've ever been ill for even a week and a half, you know how seedy it makes you feel to wear that first-thing-in-the-morning face and hairdo day after day. Even a gravely ill patient can honestly yearn to "look nicer," and an artful repair job on straggly hair and chipped nails can do wonders for sagging spirits. If the hospital itself does not have such portable service available, nurses or volunteers can surely steer you to an outside beautician who has special skills in working with patients.

The physical therapy people can be consulted for recommendations about a masseuse. A massage doesn't have to be strenuous. It can be tailored to a patient's condition, limited to legs, neck, shoulders, or even just feet, depending on the doctor's advice. This can be more than a gift; it can be a real blessing. Sometimes a skilled and gentle pair of hands can bring far greater relief than pain pills or muscle relaxants.

For Men Especially (but Not Exclusively)

Don't get hung up on "executive" type gifts if your hospitalized patient is a man. Shaving lotion, desk items, and leather goods are useless in a sickroom. Men enjoy small, thoughtful (even whimsical) gestures from the "outside" world as much as women do.

Consider buying a small, noiseless digital clock that glows in the dark. No matter that it may be immaterial what time it is to the patient rigidly scheduled by someone else's authority, every patient I've known wakes up saying, "What time is it?" I know one who unwittingly pulled out an I.V. as he grappled for his watch in the half-light. "The time" is solid information, and therefore, a source of comfort. It's like putting in a piece of a jigsaw puzzle . . . even though there are many other unfamiliar shapes still waiting to make trouble.

Television is a source of comfort, too, regardless of how little time your patient ever spends with the one at home. A TV Guide would be helpful, but the one for sale in the gift shop down in the hospital lobby is probably for *next* week; so bring the current issue from your own home. Do your friend the extra favor of listing the numbers of the local channels that are equivalents of those inside the Guide on an index card. (These mysterious numbers are usually printed and taped on top of the TV. Periscopes are not included, and a patient who is too ill to get up and down easily generally gives up on remembering that "5 is 27" and "4 is 13.") Bring paper clips to attach the card to the cover, so the patient can transfer the card to the next issue, and the next.

And last, consider a silly gift. I've seen a male patient as fascinated with a wind-up clown doing flips on his tray table as any little boy would be. Really! A silly little gadget can do double duty for your friend: he can hand it over to occupy an out-of-his-element male visitor. Even if you are absolutely sure that the man you need a gift for is All Grown Up and would not be a bit pleased with such nonsense, give the idea a chance anyway. You might just bring a crooked-y smile to that hospital-grim face.

Home Gifts

Once your friend is home, it's a good time for potted plants (aromatic herbs are a nice change, or forced bulbs about to bloom). Silk flowers can be a long-lasting alternative, especially in winter.

With a long-term convalescence ahead, your friend might enjoy a bird feeder hung on a tree limb within view of the window. If you get the sturdy variety that's sometimes labeled "squirrel-proof," your patient can count on watching marvelous gymnastics as the crafty little devils prove the label wrong. It isn't Radio City, but it does make an entertaining floor show for an invalid.

Along the same lines, you could try a nature magazine. I had an acquaintance once whose wheelchair outings in the park turned into adventures as he learned, from a Field Guide gift, to recognize even the most obscure trees and shrubs. It became a lifelong interest and a strong ally to his physical progress.

A friend or relative who is a long-term captive at home because of a health problem will find that just about any magazine subscription or newsletter helps cheer up the mailbox. A book review publication can be a wonderful gift for a shut-in, or a digest of detective fiction. You'll accomplish a dual goal here: you will help your friend keep in contact with the outside world, and you'll remind him or her, with each issue, of your continuing love and interest. But don't stop the "little" messages; no magazine can substitute for a personal note, no matter how short.

For anyone stuck in bed without a helping

hand always available, a perfect gift is one of those hanging organizers that look like shoe bags except for two major differences:

1) they're much smaller so they can hang down the side of a bed from a stiff flap that fits between the mattress and box springs; and

2) the pockets are different sizes. The pockets can hold glasses, comb, lotion, a paperback book— all the things that normally fall into the nearest crack.

The ones for sale are usually satiny and too expensive (usually sold in the same department as bed jackets). But a sewing machine and some bright fabric, plus nothing more elaborate than iron-on tape to fold over the raw top edges of the various compartments, could work together to make you a happy gift giver.

Other useful gift possibilities for a home newly turned into an infirmary include

-- a sturdy bed tray,

-- extra pillows,

-- a good reading light (those that clip onto a headboard or a book are especially handy),

-- a bedside pitcher,

-- a night light.

If you're talented at crafts, you couldn't find a worthier recipient for your creativity than an invalid. Here are a few craft ideas to consider:

-- decorating a small bedside wastebasket,

-- crocheting a bookmark,

-- making a pen and pencil holder for the bedside table,

-- embroidering a coaster for the patient's drinking glass,

-- dressing up a basket for cards.

Whether you simply dress up a Kleenex box with a painted plastic holder or crochet an entire afghan, your friend will delight in showing off your handiwork to visitors. It's nice to be able to show proof of someone's caring, isn't it? When you're ill and feeling less than self-assured, you can be excused for the repetition, many times a day, of "Did I show you what Julia made for me?"

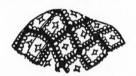

Unless the illness of your friend is relatively minor with a fairly speedy recovery time, this is going to be a difficult time for the family. You can help. Make your own Gift Certificate for pickup and delivery of laundry or dry cleaning, a take-out dinner for the family, movie tickets for the youngsters.

There's more in the following chapter on helping the family, but while you're thinking along gift lines, don't forget that the rest of your friend's household needs a pick-up as much as the one person who is the direct object of your concern. Children in particular can feel thrust into the background by an illness, and your special attention can help them through a rough time.

Is there any better way to help your friend? Bring a small gift for the resident child along with your patient-gift.

From flowers to bird-feeders to decorated Kleenex boxes, no matter what you choose, the time and attention you put in and the obvious thought and concern behind your effort is a big part of the gift. It's so easy for a person removed from the mainstream by illness to feel cut off, passed by, pushed aside in the traffic. The gift *behind* your offering is actually the important one, the message that you hold that sidelined friend in the forefront of your mind and heart.

Of course you know this already, but when you get flummoxed over finding the right gift, you can lose sight of the reason for the gift. Make yourself remember. *I want this gift to tell Sylvia how much she matters to me, how much I care.* Then you'll relax about your choices and enjoy the process. And you'll know that even if you never come up with one single perfect gift . . . even if your bows are crooked and the corners bunched, you still gave real help.

chapter four

Gifts to Do

SEVERAL YEARS AGO, when I was caring for my dearly loved friend Lee during her long, last illness, my close friend Mary gave me a gift of such enormity and good heart that it will always stand out in my mind as the hallmark of doing-gifts.

The "doing"—the pick-up and delivery of our home laundry—continued for over a year and a half, weekly, and in all kinds of weather. She made the mechanics seem casual: she would be going for herself "anyway," so she'd just swing by. It was no trouble.

No trouble! The stops took her miles out of her way with each trip, lugging baskets that I'm sure meant extra pain for her already troublesome back.

Often I didn't see Mary on either her pick-up or delivery; she always managed her stops as "background," with no expectation of coffee or a visit. I'd leave money and get change back in an envelope with the basket, along with Mrs. Johnson's yellow stick-on receipt for the ironing, all very businesslike.

I'd greet Mary every once in a while with a protest: "Mary, this is really too much!"

"No," she'd answer, her voice sharing the helpless ache for our dying Lee, "No, it's not too much. This is something I *can* do."

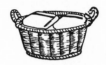

Around that same time, a large packing box bumped its way through the front door, my tiny friend Esther pushing and tugging at its bulk. Open at the top to give room to odd sizes and shapes, it spilled over with . . . paper products! There were rolls of paper towels, foil, plastic wrap, colorful paper napkins, pretty paper plates. And, you guessed it: a supply of toilet paper.

"This is the kind of thing you always run out of when you're eating on the run instead of shopping at the market," said Esther matter-of-factly as she gave the final push. She was right.

It was Esther, too, who had earlier delivered a 24-can carton of Lee's hard-to-find supplementary diet with bright green and orange yarn wrapped around it. She had somehow persuaded the dealer to mix the flavors from four other sealed cartons so that Lee wouldn't be stuck with an endless supply of strawberry if it turned out she couldn't stand the taste.

When Esther brought these things, there was no hush in tone, no effort to hide the fact that the situation was grim, but there wasn't any awkwardness about the light touch that was possible, either. She managed the perfect blend because she made what she did seem natural; she fit herself into the situation with what seemed a sixth sense: her own good sense.

Importance of Doing-Gifts

Those friends who truly mean "do" when they look for answers to "If there's anything I can do" are the family's salvation when someone needs constant care. Whatever size the illness, whether temporary or catastrophic, there are inevitable disruptions to normal daily life, and it doesn't take a genius to realize that helping the person in charge to manage those disruptions is a prime gift to any hospitalized patient or home convalescent.

Granted, the gift of your time will make the largest intrusion into your own schedule. But I don't suggest that you, like Mary, have to make a couple of hundred turns at fetch-and-carry to be of use. There are dozens of lesser, more easily managed variations on that theme. Here, even more than with other gifts, the trick is to think yourself into someone else's skin — not just shoes. Shoes aren't enough.

I know this because I've had the good fortune to have several friends with the knack of appearing at just the right moment to wave away a nagging gotta-get-to chore. There have been times when, confronting a list of trivial jobs that in my state might as well have been titled "move these mountains," I've thought, "Okay. That's it. I give up," only to have one of these genies take over and keep me intact for another day.

When I'd ask, incredulously, "How did you ever think of doing *THAT!*" the answer was always, "I figured what would help me most if I were where you are."

If I were where you are.

That's the starting point that gave Mary and Esther such standout solutions. These two friends *had* been where I was — faced with serious illnesses that compounded their responsibilities enormously, and weariness beyond what the word spells.

But I don't think one has to have experienced a similar situation first hand to be able to sense both what to do to ease another's load, and how to go about it. If you think about your own household routine for a moment, and then throw in something else that would keep you one hundred percent occupied, physically and emotionally, for at least a third of your waking hours, you'll have a fair idea of what a serious illness can mean in practical terms.

You'll realize, for example, that washing your car would have no claim on your leftover energy.

The same with cleaning out your refrigerator.

Picture yourself dragging in after long hours of shepherding your patient through fourteen different lab tests for everything from blood gases to follow-my-finger-left-to-right. How could you ever tackle an unpleasant chorus of nuisance jobs like these?

Mowing the lawn.

Picking up an appliance left for repairs.

Changing burned-out lightbulbs.

Watering the houseplants.

Now add the ingredient I call The Last Straw. The Last Straw works like this: You're somehow getting through household management, which we all know isn't a breeze at the best of times, when, out of the blue, comes an ill-tempered little gnome.

Oh, you've got a moment? Let's see what I can come up with!

He has lots to choose from. Car licenses *always* expire, library books come due, the washing machine breaks, the dog needs a distemper booster, or Junior suddenly remembers he signed up to bring twelve dozen brownies to the drama club bake sale. An illness attracts glitches the way a new white blouse attracts spills.

And in case you think such minor matters as these become irrelevant when there's a crisis going on, consider the following corollary to The Last Straw.

One of the things every patient I've known can still do perfectly, no matter how ill, is *WORRY*. Worry is such a rude companion that it doesn't even require you to be completely awake to nag at you. When you're incapacitated, worry magnifies the most insignificant concerns. You're liable to sit bolt upright in the middle of the night with a sudden flash: *I've forgotten to pay the newspaper carrier!*

I've known patients who've worked themselves into tears over some trifle that you'd expect to pale by comparison to open-heart surgery or a biopsy:

I never returned the pan I borrowed from Debbie!

I haven't sent Joe Neal his graduation card!

How could taking back a cake pan possibly weigh as heavily on a patient's mind as the sight of plasma dripping from a plastic bag into her arm? The truth is that Order on the Home Front is often a larger source of anxiety to a sick person than it has any right to be, than it would be during normal times even.

Maybe this imbalance serves a purpose. Maybe it drives a patient to get well, get up, take over the reins again. In any case, the situation gives you as friend a place to step in, a reason to *know* that your handling of a chore as minor as bringing in the newspaper on a daily basis can make a real contribution to a patient's well being. He or she won't want you to deliver it to the hospital bedside. It's getting it out of the yard that helps.

Knowing what you know of your friend's household, take a close look at that picture in your mind's eye.

Make a Plan

Once you find a place to fit yourself in with *this is something I CAN do,* then decide how to go about it. Decide how to take positive action to see your chore through from start to finish. This is important because your follow-through can make all the difference in how successful you are.

Compare these two versions of the same offer:

Betty Lou calls her friend Sally, housebound on crutches for six weeks.

"Sally, dear," she says, "I've been so worried about your not being able to get around, and I was wondering if sometime you might want me to do some errands for you. Or something."

Pause for Sally to convey her gratefulness.

"I know I'm hard to get, but keep trying!"

I don't know that you'll agree, but I think Sally could be forgiven for reading the offer as not altogether genuine . . . or heartfelt.

Now consider this version:

"I'm going to be out running errands tomorrow afternoon," says Betty Lou this time, "and I'd love to include yours. Can I do your grocery shopping or pick up your cleaning? I'm planning to come by with some of our prize tomatoes, anyway. You could give me a list?"

This new Betty Lou is clearly ready and willing; better yet, she has figured out the logistics so that it's easy as a checkmark for Sally to accept. *That's* positive action!

Here's another example. This note was stuck under my windshield wiper:

> *Good morning! Please leave a spare set of keys in your mailbox when you're done for today, and I'll get the car washed this evening. I'll return it by 8 p.m. and leave it locked. Keys in the glove box. Hope it'll add some shine to your tomorrow!*

What a joysome note to get! What a lift! My car had gone to seed during the days and days of back-and-forthing to the hospital, the way all cars do. They fill with fast-food crumbs and paper coffee cups, tissue paper and tracked-in mud (medical centers never seem to have "finished" their parking lots!). There had been times when I'd have given up my lunch money for a month to have a clean car again, but I couldn't give up the time. And part of the pure pleasure of this gift was its decisiveness, its take-charge attitude. If the note writer had said something less purposeful, something like "I'd like to get your car washed for you. How do you want me to handle it?," it's quite likely that the undertaking would have bogged down right there.

It may take some pulling and tugging at first to get your friend to lean on you and let you do unpretty chores. With doing-gifts you may have to take the risk of being just a little bossy, less polite and tentative than you might be in a normal social situation. If you can find the right mixture of light-but-insistent, your friend will feel not only comfortable about accepting, but warm and well cared for.

How to Begin

Try, for example, one of these "light entrees," maybe attached in note form to a bloom from your garden and left by your friend's front door or under a windshield wiper:

I'm yours tomorrow afternoon. No job too small.

Make my day — give me an errand tomorrow. (Your phone.) Instructions happily received after 6 p.m. tonight.

Handyman at your beck and call . . . in my jeans. (Your phone.) If it's heavy stuff, my Atlas, Jr., wants in on it, please.

Please leave your grocery list in your mailbox tomorrow morning. Delivery time from me: 4 p.m.

Willing worker desires mending, laundry, ironing. Available Mon., Wed., Fri., morning or afternoon, 1-3 hours. P.S. I'm good.

It's a good idea to include a small offering like the flower or a basket of strawberries with your message. Then the recipient can feel natural about calling to thank you, and when you repeat your offer, can feel natural about taking you up on it. Once you've gotten your foot in the door and made your honest willingness apparent, it will become easier and easier for your friend to accept your ongoing help without the nagging concern that it's too much to ask.

Car care is a great entry level chore because it's practically always needed.

Pets and plants need your help too, especially pets. If you're an animal lover, you'll know how they're thrown by a change in routine. They cannot understand, and they deserve any extra attention a qualified friend can give. You could walk the dog, providing it knows you, or simply give it your love and attention for a few minutes a day. One of my own saviors was Dee, a fellow park-walker who took over walking my dachshunds when I was ill, and took away a big chunk of worry —mine, and I'm sure, theirs.

You could offer transportation for other members of the family. When there are children, school rides may well be taken care of (but maybe not), but what about music lessons, baseball practice, the dentist? You could offer your services as chauffeur one afternoon a week or for one particular run.

If you have been given the go-ahead for the grocery shopping, you could take the offer a step further by making a master list so that the person-in-charge could simply check off the items needed. If you intend to do the shopping on an ongoing basis, you might want to pick up a key to the house and get it duplicated so you can put the groceries away, too. That solves the problem of timing if there are perishables on the list and a largely absentee family. Again, if you have thought yourself into your friend's skin, you'll know that this is not intrusion, but initiative.

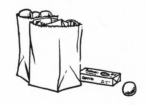

Relief for the Caregiver

If the patient is in the hospital, offer to sit the house for a morning or afternoon. It's a great boon for the person-in-charge of Home to know that you will be there on a given day. That makes possible delivery dates, repair calls, pick up from cleaners or UPS.

When the patient is at home, you can give the caregiver a great gift of time by offering to sit with the patient for a few hours at a time, taking care of basic needs. Many times this requires no more than your reassuring presence and companionship.

If you're in any doubt about your ability to handle situations that may come, *ask*. Too often, friends regard care of an invalid as too fraught with medical complexities for a "layman." High-tech hospital equipment can foster that mystique.

But for long stretches of time, most patients who are stabilized and comfortable require nothing more specialized from a friend-attendant than help to the bathroom or getting propped up for eating. Someone must be there, true. But being that same someone twenty-four hours a day is terribly demanding. If you are the special friend who can put patient care on your list of ways to help, you will be giving a *Big Help* indeed.

Even if sitting with the patient is not appropriate, you could coordinate with someone who *is* spelling the person-in-charge and arrange for one of that person's visits to tie in with your gift of a

-- theatre ticket,

-- manicure,

-- long walk together,

-- golf game,

-- gallery tour,

-- concert.

It's your initiative that's important. Too often those bearing the brunt of patient care cast themselves in such a supporting role that the clear need to "get out" once in a while is either overlooked altogether, or it is used up in some related effort.

"I'll just run down to the pharmacy and refill these prescriptions while Jennifer's with her father.

Running errands is *not* a time out. What you as the gift-giver can do—with careful planning and a healthy nudge— is to provide the kind of respite that refills energy and spirit.

You'll run into resistance: "I don't have time." "I just don't feel like going out."

Persist. If, in years to come, you hear, "I'd have managed fine during Ed's illness if only Julie hadn't forced me to go to the art museum with her that day," then you can send me this page. I'll eat it. Remember, "If I were where you are" gives you the advantage of knowing when to dig in your heels. This business of prying a weary friend away from details of illness for a few hours is one of those heel-digging times.

Help with Correspondence

Offer to write proxy notes. These can be thank-you's for cards and gifts the patient has received or progress reports for family and close friends out of town.

Sometimes writing notes can be a dreaded chore for a weak patient or run-ragged family. But if they can make you a quick list that identifies each gift with a giver's name, and provide names and addresses of those who should be kept abreast of the patient's health or progress, then you can take on the task.

Your notes should be simple, brief, and businesslike.

> *Cheryl asked me to pass along to*
> *you her thanks for the* _____.
> *As you can imagine, she's not up*
> *to writing yet, but at last report she*
> *was* _____.

Include only what you *know* to be true about Cheryl's condition, and resist the temptation to editorialize, as in "Of course, I don't think those doctors know what they're talking about." Remember that you're writing not as you, but on the patient's behalf.

You could certainly offer to take care of other miscellaneous correspondence as well. Write the checks to pay the bills, for example, so that only a signature is needed. Or tackle filling in the insurance forms — always a tedious and time-consuming chore. Handle invitations, renewals, and requests for donations. A personal secretary may be exactly what your friend needs right now.

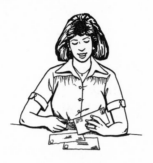

Researching Help

If you're well-organized and competent at research, offer to make yourself a resource person.

If, for instance, a long convalescence at home is involved, the family will need to gather information on home health-care equipment, nursing services, possibly even modifications to the home such as a wheelchair ramp or bathtub bars. You can put together a list of agencies and contact people who can provide assistance and support in all aspects of home care — teaching the family how to lift and bathe the patient, for example. Other agencies provide services such as respite care, housekeeping help, physical therapy, nutrition counseling, even telephone reassurance calls.

Sometimes such information is readily available through the hospital, but there are still hours of homework to be done on the telephone, comparing prices and ascertaining exactly what is covered by insurance and what isn't. You can help further by getting personal recommendations from former clients of those agencies — a job that takes more time and often involves lengthier conversations than any family member can spare right now.

When your patient is going home to be cared for round-the-clock by a family member who insists he or she can "manage without help," compile that list of recommended nurses anyway.

You *KNOW* that if 24-hour care is needed for very long, the job will be too much for one person. If you can hand over a ready-made list of names, with phone numbers and sources of your information, with a casual, "This is for you to keep in case you do need nursing help," you will make it easier, if that time does come, for your friend to get over what might otherwise have remained a big emotional hurdle. Your list will be like money in the bank, a comfort as well as an actual resource.

Helpful Neighbors

Now let's say that you're a near neighbor. Not a good friend, maybe, but friendly enough that when you look across the street and see Milly Thompson's car pull in late night after night, and you hear that George is in intensive care, the situation tugs at you.

Maybe you've been talking with other neighbors, all of you wishing there were something you could do without butting in.

There almost certainly is. Here's just a sample of things you or the group of you could offer to take on:

Accept deliveries (Milly can leave a note on her door).

Shut windows in case of rain.

Turn on and off sprinklers.

Clear the walk of snow.

Take trash out to the curb on garbage day.

Turn on the driveway light.

Turn on an indoor light at night, draw shades, adjust the thermostat. (Offer to make a duplicate key.)

Bring things to the hospital. You, or another close neighbor who's home much of the time, could give Milly your telephone number and schedule, saying you'll be available if she needs anything brought to the hospital on short notice.

Again — and to me this is the key to the whole doing-gift strategy — the way to do Milly the most good is to organize the effort and present it with an imaginary ribbon around it. Don't wait to be asked. You can consult with Milly, sure, but when you do, have a positive idea in mind, offer your suggestions, and then reinforce them with your obvious intention to follow through without further ado or daily thanks. And leave it at that. Don't let Milly think that state-of-George reports are a prerequisite for your readiness to help.

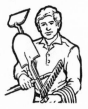

I did say earlier that I'd include some classic "how not to" examples, and here is one of them. It concerns a one-time next door neighbor I shall call Eunice.

Eunice was a semi-invalid herself, or at least she didn't have much to do. What Eunice was good at was keeping a watch on the neighborhood from her kitchen window. She rarely missed a coming or going, day or night. And what Eunice offered me during a family member's hospitalization was exactly that: she would "keep an eye" on the house for me while I spent days and evenings at the hospital, in case anything unusual happened.

"Please do," I told her, thinking that it never hurts to have someone keeping track of your empty house. Unfortunately, the only unusual activity Eunice had to report upon was mine.

"Susan!" the voice on the other end of the phone would say, whatever the hour that I had finally straggled in.

"I just saw you drive up. How *is* Lee?"

I can only think that Eunice was a closet ambulance-chaser and that this situation was the answer to her prayers. In return for doing what she did all the time anyway, Eunice got a direct hotline to an actual emergency situation. I'm ashamed to say that it took me a long time to catch on, and even longer to get up the gumption to tell her I was simply too tired to give her details.

For the Patient at Home

There are a number of gifts-you-can-do that fall under the heading of Making Life Easier once the patient is actually at home.

Some of them involve a purchase. When that's the case, the matter of who is to bear the expense should be discussed ahead of time. Your gift is in making the arrangements, locating the item, seeing to the installation. If you *can* take on the financial burden, great; if not, there's nothing wrong with saying, "I can't afford to actually get you a _____. But if it's something you would like to have, I'll look into it and make all the arrangements."

An FM call system, for example, can be a real boon in a sickroom.

Rental of a water cooler for the patient's room is often a good idea. (Many patients are instructed to drink as much water as they can possibly hold.)

A telephone with an automatic dial function is a wonderful aid for a convalescent who likes to make frequent calls but whose fingers can't do the dialing.

Remote control for the television can be added on. Many patients watch a great deal even if they didn't before, and they like the independence of not having to ask for an on-off or channel change.

A small table on wheels that can hold correspondence, puzzles, books, or lists of all kinds, and that can be placed in front of any chair any time, is extremely handy.

There are a number of kitchen aids to help a person who is alone a great deal but not functioning perfectly. Just think how much bending and tugging a step-on garbage can saves, for example.

And one of my own favorites in the Making Life Easier category is an eight to ten foot expandable telephone cord for the kitchen phone, allowing a less-than-sturdy person access to a chair after she's answered the phone. (It also allows a busy person-in-charge to do more than one thing at once — a real necessity.)

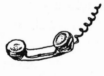

Knowing your friend's particular condition, you can think of other nonmedical conveniences. For help, search your mind for the names of friends or acquaintances who have been housebound with ailments similar to your friend's. Call those valuable contacts and ask what came in handiest.

Anybody who's ever had the use of only one

hand for any length of time, for instance, can pass on tricks you never could have imagined. One friend of mine whose broken wrist was in a cast figured out an ingenious way to butter her own toast. She got her husband to put six nails into a short piece of board. The nails were long enough for the points to extend about an inch beyond the wood. The gadget made a much better anchor for buttering toast than her elbows had!

It's amazing how often a bright idea for some simple procedure can become a real lifesaver — or psyche saver. Sure, that husband would have buttered the toast for her every morning. But it's very hard for most patients to get out of their usual role, to have to be helped all the time, to try to fit requests into a convenient time slot for the one who's helping. Finding the solutions other patients have come up with to solve the daily problems of managing independently could lead to an invaluable gift.

The "doing" kind of gift is not easy. Its cost is high in time, patience, interest, understanding, and imagination.

If your own schedule and capacity make it too difficult for you to "do" a gift instead of buying one, you shouldn't feel defensive about it. You should take the pleasure that is your due in arranging for a dozen long-stemmed American beauties, or even six. But when you *can* slip into the right niche at the right time, when you can be sure that your actions brought your friend an hour's peace of mind and pleasure, then I promise that the reward for your time and effort is deep, deep satisfaction.

chapter five

Visits

ALMOST THE FIRST question to a doctor or family member who breaks the news about illness, injury, or operation is *When can I see her?* or *Can he have visitors yet?*

We want to visit, and even when we don't totally relish the prospect, we expect it of ourselves. It doesn't seem, on the face of it, all that hard. You get in your car, drive to St. Whoever's, find a parking spot, go in and give the patient your regards, chat a while, and then you leave.

But if it's really so simple, why are you gulping a nervous gulp deep down about how that visit is going to go?

Truly, there is an art to a good visit to a patient. And guess where that buck stops? Right. With *you* alone. A successful visit certainly isn't the patient's responsibility. That's why you're feeling those doubts, however much you want to take your love in person to room 423.

Let's face it—hospital visits aren't easy. It's hard for most of us to feel comfortable and self-assured, with the right words poised on our tongues to express our caring and concern. We don't know what to expect, so how can we be sure our visit will be a pleasure for both sides, from the moment we enter the room until the patient bids us goodbye? We can only hope we'll seem confident, and that the patient will be radiant with "Please come back again!"

But in all my considerable years of visitor-watching, I've known only one person who could consistently pull off that kind of visit to patients with all kinds of illness and behavior patterns. She's also a doctor, which fact may have something to do with her effortless skill (she does get a lot of practice). The rest of us can use some help, I think, in the area of paying a visit to a very ill friend or relative.

I say "very ill" because this chapter is not about dropping in on someone who could manage open house if friends brought refreshments. We rarely need any answers about visiting a friend who has just had a baby or commiserating with a tennis partner recouping from knee surgery. These visits are no big deal; usually they're fun.

But visits to patients in critical condition are an entirely different matter. They're not fun. They often take a great deal of effort, emotional and otherwise. But they needn't be the nerve-wracking, awkward occasions that they too often become.

The guidelines that follow won't guarantee successful visits, but I hope they will ease the unsureness and prepare you to give the visit your best.

Be Prepared

Unless you operate on a different plane from most people, the first problem you'll encounter, well before opening that hospital room door, is your own nervousness and anxiety. What will your friend/aunt/uncle look like? Will s/he be terribly depressed? Will s/he really want to see you? Be confused? Easily upset? What will you talk about? What if something goes wrong while you're in the room?

There's no way to know what to expect, and so your imagination kicks into overdrive. This is the time to "take yourself in hand," as my grandmother used to say. You must turn that concern away from yourself and from what you might find, and make certain, instead, that it is focused where it belongs: on the patient. There, it can be constructive.

I've seen people behave in some very *un*constructive ways when they let their nervousness run away with them. This is what can happen:

I can still picture Marjorie, who blew into the room like a tornado and, with barely a glance at the patient, began reeling off details of her morning's shopping, last evening's cocktail party, her recent car problems . . . on and on.

To keep herself busy during her mindless monologue, Marjorie picked up and put down every item in the room—at least twice. She finished by using the patient's tiny bathroom to re-apply her own makeup. "Well," she said, when she finally ran out of steam, "you're tired, and I've got to run." And run she did.

Marjorie meant well or she wouldn't have been there. But she made the mistake of allowing her nervous energy to take control, and as a result she ignored the patient. Maybe she assumed, as some visitors do, that the patient would prefer her to pretend that nothing was wrong. The trouble with that seemingly kind but one-sided "pact" was that Marjorie made it without consulting the patient.

In actuality, this patient knew full well that she was very ill. She was also completely lucid and enjoyed conversation. She didn't need to be treated as though she were invisible, and she certainly didn't need a whirlpool of forced joviality in the room—she could have had that by turning on the TV.

Dan-from-the-office went to another extreme to cover his unsureness. He sailed in on a stream of borrowed platitudes that had nothing to do with the patient's actual condition. This pep-talker didn't seem to realize that people don't lose their distaste for insincerity just because they've lost some bodily functions.

"What a rotten break," Dan started out. "But chin up, buddy, you'll be back on your feet in no time . . . hope they're not too rough on you here . . . you do what those docs tell you . . . stiff upper lip . . . you look just great, can't believe you're sick . . . well, hang in there . . . now, if there's anything I can do . . . ."

During this non-exchange, the patient tried to play the gracious host: his poor head agreed, up and down, trying for synchronization. Actually, he would have enjoyed telling about his major progress that day, a walk down the hall and back. But Dan never asked . . . anything! The two of them never did connect because Dan was no closer to being ready to *LISTEN* than Marjorie had been.

Remember the Paul Tillich quotation, "The first duty of love is to listen"? It ought to be engraved on the mind of anyone with a very ill friend.

The third example of the emotionally non-prepared visitor is the worst, because it's hardest on the patient. Jeffrey had driven three and a half hours to pay a visit to his beloved Aunt Sarah who had suffered a stroke a month before. Aunt Sarah of the bristly temper covering a heart of honey. Aunt Sarah who had practically raised him.

With head and heart brimming with a scrapbook's worth of memories, Jeff stepped into her room . . . and froze. He gasped audibly. This tiny, frail blue-lipped figure in the bed *couldn't* be Aunt Sarah. She opened her eyes, obviously recognized him, and smiled. Jeff couldn't even begin to stifle a sob. He ran. Poor both of them!

These are examples of unproductive visits that sap a patient's strength, and they do nothing for the visitor either. What's missing is not the element of caring. But each visitor lacked the kind of mental preparation that I think has to be a part of any visit to a critically ill patient.

Making Your Visit Work

The prime ingredient, the factor with which all visits to critically ill patients must be layered, is *kindness*. Not politeness. Not social graces or good manners, and not the art of exchanging pleasantries. These social virtues we have been taught since childhood are for visits between persons on equal footing. You and your patient are not on equal footing. *YOU* are in control. The tone and the duration of the visit are up to you.

The patient is pinned helplessly to the bed, subject to your scrutiny. The sickroom is, for now, an arena for the patient's life. Since you are in the captain's seat, you need to be ready to take unusual measures and make allowances that could be strange in a normal social context. If you pretend that this is an everyday visiting situation and that your patient will benefit if you act as though the two of you were sitting down for a drink, it won't work — because it isn't true. Telling your friend he looks great won't help anything, in most cases, because that isn't true either. The *only* thing that will work in this inequitable situation is honest kindness.

What is the kindest thing you can do? Before you visit, you need to think out the answer, walking quietly in your mind through the probable strengths and weaknesses of your patient as you put evidence together from all possible sources. The results of your mental measurements can vary enormously. Let me give two examples:

One visitor, a lifelong friend of my mother, sat without word or movement for three or four hours at each visit, close up to Mother's bed, communicating strength and peace to her dying friend by holding her hand. As I came and went, I, too, felt the balm of that benediction-without-voice.

And then there was the radiant young girl who brought her fiance a basket of foolish food and bright-checked tablecloth. She had managed the necessary permissions from doctors and staff, and now she was intent on creating brightness, even gaiety, with a shared-memory picnic in the hospital room of her heart's love, now ravaged by cancer — an old, old man at twenty.

From one I learned about how kind stillness can be (though not necessarily three or four hours of it!). From the other, I found out that the brave kindness in what seems like an impossible gesture can make more sense sometimes than any other medicine.

Where can you get your ideas?

They have to come from you and from what you know about your patient. Ask yourself what the patient can possibly react to, can possibly "use" when so much energy is gone. Please don't try to duplicate either of the examples that had such a profound effect on me. The important thing to remember from them is that these two visitors, separated by more than forty years in age, allowed their own special awareness to lead them. You can do it too.

This kindness, as you see, comes in such different forms that you might want to think out your visit in stages. That process can give you a sense of order to fall back on. Sometimes, for me, having made a set of procedures to follow is like having an imaginary safety net underneath when I actually get there: if I have that net, I won't need it!

The following can be your outline for a visit. I hope you'll feel comfortable about tossing out the divisions and concentrating on the content because, above all, kindness is flexible.

Before Visiting

Do your homework and try to get a realistic idea of what to expect. Plan your visit, if possible, with the family member who is in charge.

What time of day is usually the patient's best?

What is his or her general condition?

Is there anything you should be particularly aware of?

The person-in-charge will appreciate your consideration in asking, even when the patient is capable of answering the questions, because it is that person who probably bears the brunt of a bad night when the patient is overtired or stretched too thin.

And no matter how positive an outlook you're given, be aware that you may catch the patient at an off-time and find him listless, confused, irritable, or in more pain than usual. Illness brings big ups and downs. If you're mentally prepared for that possibility, you won't be caught. You'll merely adjust your expectations.

A few DON'Ts should go into your planning:

Don't ever go to visit with the slightest sign of a cold, even if you're sure it's "just allergies."

Don't take the children on either a home or hospital visit unless the patient specifically asks for them. (Even though hospitals aren't so tough about children anymore, you'd better ask to be sure that it's O.K. to bring them.)

Don't go on your lunch break if it means you'll have to sit in the room eating your sandwich.

Don't, in general, plan to just drop by, even though it's obvious your friend isn't going anywhere. Call to ask. Give advance notice.

And *do* plan to limit your visit to thirty minutes at the most.

Be Prepared for Snags

In planning a hospital visit, there are a few possible hurdles that you should be ready to encounter.

First, though, if you're uneasy at the stodgy, authoritarian picture you hold in your mind of hospitals, you can take heart in this: they are altogether different from the way they used to be. The personnel seem genuinely willing to let visitors use their own good judgment about whether to visit, when, and for how long.

No one asks "What are you doing here?" with a menacing, beady eye any more. And though visiting hours are still posted, the signs often seem mainly to be an excuse for someone to practice skills with black ink and stencils. If, because of your schedule, you and your patient need to bend those hours for your visit, the nurses will doubtless cooperate.

But if you arrive at your patient's room, announced or not, to find a NO VISITORS sign on the door, it means no, none, not any, nobody.

"Why, I've been like a mother to him!" or "She and I go back as far as kindergarten!" or "I'm sure he's expecting me!" are not credible excuses for ignoring the sign. The patient is not to be disturbed. It's that simple.

Your best course is to leave a note at the nurse's station for delivery later. If the nurses aren't busy, they may be able to explain the tie-up to you and suggest a better time. Then you can mention in your note when you'll be back.

The second possible hurdle is your arriving to find someone else in the room. It may be a doctor, a nurse, even a mutual friend with whom you might enjoy sharing this visit. Yet I recommend that you back out, smiling, without discussion, and find a chair down the hall. A discussion would only yield up the information that either the person is "about ready" to leave, or that the patient wants you to stay, *wants* you to.

If the someone else is a staff member, the patient surely won't benefit from your presence during medical procedures. And nurses and doctors may not take the initiative in asking a visitor to leave. They have no idea whether the visitor is just an acquaintance from the patient's apartment building or near-and-dear Aunt Effie, just arrived from Istanbul.

Too, the patient may not feel up to requesting privacy It's hard to say, "Could you please go away for a few minutes?" Consider, too, the possibility that the patient has been waiting all day to ask the doctor questions about the illness, or the medication, or some new symptoms.

Better all the way around if you state briefly,

"It's Emma Harris, and I'll wait in the hall," and then ease yourself right out. If the nurse/doctor procedure lasts longer than you can wait, tell your patient quickly that you will call later that evening or come back tomorrow.

Do show enough kindness to specify your next contact and soften your friend's disappointment; your own can be assuaged by knowing that after so much visiting or handling, your bowing out gracefully is undoubtedly right for the patient.

If the someone else is another visitor, I suggest you don't risk overloading your patient with a multiple visit. Again, say that you will wait in the hall. If the other visitor doesn't pick up the hint and leave after ten minutes or so, go on in and suggest a trade-off: "Can I borrow the bedside chair for just a few minutes?"

The third hurdle is fortunately rare, but when it presents itself, it can be a shock. You open the door to the room and find the bed empty! Your patient is doubtless in some lab or other, but your first reaction gives you no time to think. Your heart leaps to your throat.

Since you know now that it can happen, you can save your blood-pressure surge for something else. And if it does happen, my advice is to leave instead of waiting. Think of the patient's probable weariness once returned to the room, and save your visit for another day.

If you're from out of town, or if you know ahead

of time that you can't visit again for weeks, then you'd better go to the hospital prepared for possible hurdles. Take along *War and Peace!*

Beginning the Visit

For those who flounder when visiting sick relatives or friends, the beginning is especially hard. I have a good solution: take some little hand offering —a dogwood twig, a bunch of autumn leaves tied with yarn, a shiny piece of fruit, a treat to share. This isn't a real gift; it's more of a disposable swatch from the outside world to give your entrance a kind of happy flourish, and to give your hands something to do. I know from experience that advancing through that hospital door can be easier with an auxiliary "hello" in one hand. Comments on your offering will give you and your patient a launching point for conversation, and give you time to get your cues for the visit.

Two guidelines will start you on the right track:

First, adapt your tone of voice and the speed with which you speak to the amount of light in the patient's room.

If the shades are drawn against daylight, speak softly and slowly. If it's evening and there's only a dim baseboard light, forget about the jolly banner you were going to hang. It may fit before you leave, but don't jump right in unless you've come into a room full of sunshine or with the overhead lights on.

Second, be sure your friend knows who you are.

Make eye and hand contact, right away. Don't assume that a long-term friendship can automatically prod an illness-clouded mind. Walk easily to the bed, lean over so that your voice will be distinct and say something like, "It's Louise, dear." Or your whole name. Better to have the patient laugh with "Well I hardly expected an introduction!" than to risk her anxiousness and confusion when she can't make the long-known face fit a name.

If you'd rather, work your name into a quick comment, like "There was no place to park, but I found a spot over on Grand and I just said, Jane Clark, it wouldn't hurt you a bit to walk!" This self-identification isn't belittlement in any way. It's kindness.

Touch your patient's hand or arm, gently. If it feels comfortable to you, let your hand continue resting on your friend's as you talk. The physical contact will give true comfort, if you can be natural about it.

As you're beginning to settle in, there are often other clues you can pick up that will help with your visit. Are there books beside the bed? Good. Your patient may enjoy having you read out loud. Is there a wheelchair? Your friend may appreciate your taking her for a walk.

Check the equipment in the room, the location

of the call button, the telephone, your friend's eye-glasses and water glass. Be aware, so that if a need comes up during your visit, you'll be able to help— easily, quickly, naturally.

I've actually seen visitors stay comfortably seated, asking "Can I help?" when there's a spill (it's not easy drinking in a prone position), or a sudden wild look of nausea (common after surgery), or a tangled I.V. cord that needs a nurse's attention. Being prepared in case will help you keep from under- or overreacting. If it's a little problem, you can manage. If it's bigger, you can get help. Help is not far away, and you won't add to the problem by indecision, or "where's your call button?," or worse: shouting down the hall.

After your greeting, don't sit down in a chair that's across the room and two towering I.V.'s away from the patient, just because that's where it happens to be. Pull the chair close enough to the bed that you can face your friend and talk without raising your voice. If the hospital room is shared, ask if the patient would like you to pull the curtain for privacy.

Take your coat off and park your belongings beside the chair, not on your lap, so you won't seem poised to fly off to your next appointment. And *not* on the patient's bed. Yes, it does happen, though I have no idea why anyone would think a patient would enjoy sharing leg space with a large purse. Settle yourself quickly, and prepare to give your friend the benefit of your calm, centered attention for the next twenty minutes or so.

Mid-Visit

"It's good to be with you," you seem to say, as you sit down with a smile, a light touch, a sigh of pleasure. Make your tone positive, and let your openers give the patient an opportunity to talk to you about what's going on.

You might ask a question or two about the hospital routine.

> *Tell me, is it true they wake you up at dawn for breakfast?*
>
> *Not getting fond of orange jello, are you?*
>
> *Are the nurses always this nice?*

Or something like,

> *How do you manage that smile! I'd think you'd growl at anyone coming through the door when you have to be strung up like that!*

Or a sympathetic,

> *This isn't much fun for you, is it?*

By the response, or lack of it, you will pick up signals about whether your friend wants to talk about the illness. Many patients do, and it's good for them, regardless of the conventional wisdom that says it's better to avoid painful topics and talk about the weather instead.

When your friend does want to talk, you should become a total and dedicated audience, listening and commiserating, and *not* talking about your own or others' similar experiences and operations. Don't offer opinions on "What I would do" unless you are asked. Instead, *LISTEN.* Give the patient time to order his thoughts or rest between sentences, without hurrying the conversation. This is one of those areas where you vary your "normal" social patterns. Slow down to your friend's pace.

If your friend doesn't feel like talking at all, you'll know that from the dead-end, monosyllabic responses to your first questions. You have several choices of other ways to offer your companionship. You can do the talking yourself, and if, for example, you begin an anecdote about the office and get a spark of interest at the punchline, you'll know that's a good route. If you're a passable storyteller (not jokes), this can be a wonderful visit.

Another way to spend the visit is with a shared activity. You could watch a television show together, listen to music, take a walk down the corridor if permitted, work on a puzzle, or play a game of cards. You could read aloud from that book you noticed when you sat down.

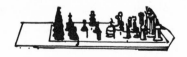

Remember, you're the one in charge— but it's not the same as with doing-gifts for the patient's family, where you insist on your willingness. Here you offer your suggestions, and you make it easy on the patient to pass. If the response is, "I don't think so, not right now," it's better not to push, even when you're sure that activity is good for idle minds and bodies.

Don't be concerned that your visit is a waste if you get no conversation going, no matter what you try. You can still fall back on choice number three, and it's a fine one: a deliberate quiet, during which you bring out your handiwork or reading, or simply sit with the patient. Your friend won't think you're a piece of furniture. You've already shown your interest and given him a wide open invitation. If he suddenly feels more talkative or energetic, he'll feel perfectly comfortable in changing the mood.

Lee, who herself was most voluble on her good days, said at one point, "Please ask Edith to come back. She is so quiet. She's just there when I open my eyes." Granted, she was very ill when she said that, but I've learned that even not-so-ill patients can enjoy a whole afternoon of wordless companionship.

If you have a horror of silence left over from that piano recital in seventh grade when you got stuck in the middle of your number, force yourself past it. Don't panic! Get up quietly and go to the window. Or sit where you are and let the patient know you appreciate the chance to share this wordless communication between friends. After all, the silence itself was not responsible for those remembered agonies. It just got left when everything that should have happened didn't. Silence itself can be beautiful, as in church where we don't question it, or as between two people sharing a sunrise.

What if all is going well and then suddenly there's an intrusion: a doctor or nurse, an aide, another visitor? This isn't likely when you're visiting the patient at home, because the family will probably run interference, but in the hospital it's common. It's up to you to put the patient first.

If all that's going to happen is a temperature and blood pressure reading, you can simply move out of the way and keep quiet. (Although a good RN can time 120/80 with someone right there beating on a snare drum, there's no point in making her prove it.) But preparation for changing of bandages, treating sutures, abdominal palpations, or a start on personal questions ought to be a signal for you to step outside without fanfare and wait in the hall. Your best bet is to ask the nurse, right at the beginning: "Is this going to be X-rated for the likes of me?" You're the one who can ensure against any possible embarrassment, so you should. You might be surprised to know how many visitors thoughtlessly stay and gape.

If another guest comes in and starts to make him- or herself comfortable, there's only one sure answer. Contain your resentment, rise, and leave as soon as possible. Again, kindness to the patient is the measure. Down the hall an entire battalion may be throwing a surprise party for a patient just as sick as yours, and here you're making yourself leave just because one other guest has been inconsiderate enough not to wait. But you can take comfort in knowing that your actions can't possibly set your patient back, whereas those partygoers may leave the whole nursing staff groaning, "Those were *friends?*"

Another reason to cut your visit short is a signal or signals from the patient. Your antennae will improve with experience in visiting, but even a novice should notice telltale signs of fatigue and strain, like sudden restlessness, feet thrashing under the covers, decreasing voice level, slowing of speech, aimless plucking at the covers, maybe an erratic punching of pillows and an inability to find a comfortable position.

When any such behavior shows up, you should leave. Forget the thirty minutes. Go right to "end of visit" in your pre-planned mental outlines, and make yours a pleasant leave-taking before your stay outlives its purpose.

End of Visit

Finales to sickroom visits can suffer the same awkwardness we find at the "good-bye" stage of any function, no matter how much we practiced "thank you, I had a very nice time" as children. A smooth combination of rising with a smile and a pat on the hand, then saying "I'll go along now," or "I'll be going now and I'll be back next Wednesday," and then heading straight for the door is surely not a difficult feat.

But much more common is this type of scene:

The visitor handles the "I'll-be-going" part fine. Then she begins to gather up her things, barely remembering the umbrella she left hanging over the door handle. The patient begins to squirm. Then our visitor thinks of one more thing.

"Oh, I meant to give you a message from Marty . . ."

The patient squirms more (he's been waiting until the visitor leaves to call the nurse for a bed pan and pain medication).

"Now I really am leaving," announces the visitor, with another wave and a blown kiss. "I'll just put a little more water in this vase for you on my way out. Oh, let me tell you a trick I have for keeping tulips fresh . . . ."

The patient clenches his teeth. The visitor dithers like someone at a Christmas party trying to save the used ribbons. Finally she backs toward the door with a last comment or two, and reaches it just in time to collide with the supper tray bearer pushing in. I've seen it happen more than once.

When you've said you're leaving, do leave. Without making your patient nervous with a lot of false starts, returns, reminders, last-minute advice, and straightening up. And walk to the door facing it, for three good reasons: hospital doors are totally noiseless for the sake of patients, they open inward, and nobody knocks.

Earlier I talked about the immeasurable importance of support from friends during a critical illness. Friends bring life, laughter, solace, and a feeling of continuity with the outside world. Never can these be conveyed more warmly than during a face-to-face, sit-down visit. If visiting sick friends is always on the top of your agenda, then you know already the pleasure of giving a lift to a loved one by your sheer presence. But if you've always thought that visits to sick people are a bad idea, or if you've always felt you *should* visit, but you've stayed off Hospital Hill because you didn't think you'd do very well, you may be missing something very precious that you are capable of giving.

I hope this chapter has given you the assurance to try. I hope it's changed your notion that you have to be an entertainer or a great talker to be a good visitor. But however you decide, do think about it as a new subject. It is good for us all to challenge our mind sets from time to time.

Otherwise, how would anyone ever try yogurt?

chapter six
Food Flair

YOU NEED NO SPECIAL qualifications. Whether you're a whiz with a whisk, at home with *parboil* and *flambe,* or whether you're barely on speaking terms with Tbsp. and tsp., you can enjoy the possibilities of "food flair" when you have a friend or relative who is ill or coping with grief.

The great thing about food as a way to help is that there are literally hundreds of ways to go, from a basket of fruit to a full-blown hot meal for the family with a week's worth of leftovers. And there is never a need to question whether taking food is the right choice, the tactful and considerate thing to do. It always is. Families never outgrow their need for food, not even when shopping is impossible and cooking no pleasure. Food is simply a can't-miss way of taking care of friends during hard times.

Food has a special place on my own mental

mantelpiece for gifts that I have been most grateful for. If the lasting impression they have made on me is any indicator, your efforts are going to be remembered — much longer than a frilly bathrobe or pot of mums — as shining examples of "what my friends did." Doesn't that make the trouble seem worthwhile?

You'd think the taste of food, not to mention the looks, wouldn't begin to compute when I was one hundred percent involved in the situation at hand. Yet how well I remember that first slippery-cold taste of ice cream after a tonsillectomy, the homemade lemon meringue that went down when nothing else would, the steaming lasagna brought by a neighbor when Mother was in the hospital! And nothing has ever made me feel quite as cared for as coming home from a long bedside stint at the hospital to one of my friend Frances' carefully wrapped and hand-delivered meals-for-one, complete with fresh out-of-season raspberries.

Before I trot out my favorite ideas and recipes, I'd better acknowledge that I'm no Julia Child, or even a poor relation. My kitchen skills might (generously) be described as basic. Normally I pay about as much attention to fixing and eating food as I do to polishing the silver. I'm always forgetting to eat and wondering why I feel so limp, and even then I'd rather wolf down a peanut butter sandwich than savor a salade nicoise. You might think, then, that I'd make a pretty poor authority on the subject.

Not so. My experience as a guinea pig is — thanks to the friends you'll hear about in this chapter — extensive. And actually, my very nonchalance might qualify me as an ideal judge. If something in the food line makes *me* sit up and take notice, it has to be special.

In this chapter, I've put together a sampling of food ideas that either dented my own customary indifference or made their mark with one specific friend or another when *they* needed it. Each one is "field-tested." I know they work at the eating end. Along with the recipes, I've added suggestions for the "flair" part of food flair: the big and small ways of enhancing food gifts so they'll come off to your, and your patient's, best advantage.

Planning

First, though I know I've tooted this planning-and-timing horn before, please don't run off while I put in one more pitch for that major aid-to-success. Try to spread out the dates for delivery of food gifts and coordinate with other friends if possible.

A kitchen table full of edible wonders that come all at once can surely boost the family's morale. But the pile-up also creates unnecessary problems about what to do with it all. Stuff it into unhungry mouths? Freeze it? (A shame when those carefully-chosen ingredients would be so much better fresh.) Share it with neighbors and feel a little guilty about "all that work" going somewhere not intended? Or (groan) throw a good deal of it away and feel a lot guilty!

So please, unless your friend is otherwise friendless, wait at least a few days before preparing your dish. Give the crowd that always storms the deli their chance to fire and fall back. Reserve your own best efforts for those long, empty days to come. They'll come, indeed they will.

Another part of planning is deciding what kind of food will be most appreciated. Depending on who the recipient is, here's a basic rule of (my) thumb:

Food-gifts for hospitalized patients should be small-scale and entertaining.

Food for their families should be practical and hearty, should keep well, and should reheat easily.

And a third category, special food for special patients, should be "designer"-made, tempting while also fitting into a limited diet.

In all cases, you can avoid waste and possible embarrassment by taking care, well before you pick up your spatula, to match your recipe to the recipient.

Are family members vegetarian?

Kosher?

Trying to maintain a low-fat diet?

Is the patient forbidden cholesterol or salt?

Are there food allergies?

Giving a pot roast to a vegetarian or deviled eggs to a heart patient can turn a generous gesture into an awkward and costly mistake.

If you've done this homework and found that there *are* restrictions, label your dish "salt-free soup" or "meatless lasagna" so that nobody needs to guess.

Presentation

A final entry on your planning checklist, and a big contributor to the "flair" part of your efforts, is the presentation of your dish. In glossy food magazines, "presentation" means serving glorious meals on a glamorously-set table in your country home in the Hamptons. With candles.

Here, it means using inexpensive containers you can live without, or planning to retrieve them. Or better yet, sending your dish in a reusable refrigerator storage dish, one that you donate as part of your gift.

It means coordinating delivery arrangements in advance, and being sure to include everything necessary for enjoyment of your dish, like written instructions such as, *Warm this as is (no cover) for 25 - 30 minutes at 350 degrees —no microwave — sorry!*

It means all the little, thoughtful touches: the note saying, "No thanks necessary, just enjoy"; the jar of parmesan cheese for your spaghetti; the packet of crackers for your soup.

And—lest you think I'm touting a drab proposition—it does mean looks, too. Don't skimp on the garnish, the pretty topping, the twist of lemon that marks this dish as one of your specialties. Don't think, "This is no time to be frivolous." You'll never find a better time or a more receptive audience, no matter what the setting, for the kind of pleasure you can give with beautifully prepared food.

Let's start with food-gifts for patients, since you may be wondering what on earth I mean by "entertaining."

Food for the Hospital

For most ill patients, any food gift is a momentary diversion, more than an end in itself. Even if you've checked with the floor nurse and found that there are no dietary restrictions, you'll probably find that your patient is short on appetite, and that it makes more sense to bring a small, tantalizing offering — as a bit of fun between the morning's watery eggs and evening's gray meat — than to try to supply your friend with any of the daily minimum requirements.

Besides, probably the food will come with you attached, and if the treat can enhance your visit, it will serve a much better purpose than your bringing a big amount of something "for later."

More than once I've seen one of those towering commercial fruit baskets, all festively shrink-wrapped, just sit there on the crowded hospital dresser until the bananas turn brown. Fresh fruit is a fine idea, but these displays are often just too much. The patient doesn't want to break into all that plastic and tissue for one single apple. It just seems too difficult.

The same thing goes for oversize chocolate chip cookies or ten kinds of cheese and crackers. By day four of sharing his bed with the crumbs and his bedside table with the scarcely chipped-at cookies, your friend may begin to tire of their company. I'm not saying this quantity rule applies across the board (certainly not for a recovering patient at home with visitors), but I do want to offer alternatives for the times when flair is more important than fare.

Fruit is a happy choice, but instead of the cornucopia approach, bring a dime store vase with a "bouquet" of washed seedless grapes, which your friend can pop into her mouth while you talk. No mess, fuss, or overripe leftovers.

Try a ring of strawberries with a custard cup of powdered sugar in the center for dipping.

Or a crisp apple — peeled, cored and sliced, courtesy of you. The same patient who stares right past a whole apple for days will gobble it up delightedly in slices dusted with cinnamon sugar. (My mother practiced this nutritional sleight-of-hand on me for years, and it never failed.)

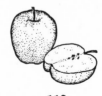

Or try fresh-squeezed orange juice. You can make it an activity by taking a tote bag with couple of oranges, your own small paring knife and a hand juicer, and produce a glass of juice right there in the room while you visit. You'll add pleasure if you make some for the person in the next bed, too, if it's a double. Just make sure there's a place to work (the bathroom sink may come in handy) and that you have a paper towel handy you can dampen to wipe up any mess. (Sweet grapefruit, peeled and sectioned, is a close runner-up.)

To go to the head of the class in Fruit Flair, freeze a half-pint container of fruit salad for forty-five minutes before you go to the hospital. Your patient, if he's like most, will enjoy a chilled fruit cup more than almost anything— *nothing* tastes so good on a dry tongue. (Bring a spoon or fork with you, or borrow one from the hospital cafeteria.)

If your friend loves pastries and you do choose baked goods, avoid being overgenerous. Estimate how long before staleness will set in, and then figure that your friend (unless he's lean and seventeen), probably won't eat more than two or three a day of, let's say, brownies. Add a couple of giveaways, and then pack your treats with either speed (a sack) or artistic additions (ribbon and box), and present it with all the flourish accorded a two-pound box of candy, without the overkill. Bring a cloth napkin for a touch of class and to act as a crumb-catcher, held up to the chin to give your patient an edge in the ongoing challenge of eating while flat on his back.

I like the "tea for two" approach to combining food and visit. It's another area where you can carve your own niche among visitors. You bring everything for this festive occasion, including the tea (Thermos or hot pot), cups, sugar, real cream in a little jar, plates and forks for whatever accompanying treat you choose. (Yes, some of that paraphernalia may be available in the hospital room, but it won't be if you're counting on it.) Individual tarts are good tea-time entertainment; so are pettits fours—bite-size cakes you can find at any French bakery.

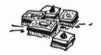

If you're feeling fancy, you might like to try my friend Frances' favorite formula for a really special bedside teatime: Madeleines Cordon Bleu. Anybody who's read Proust ought to try them once in a lifetime. Don't worry, the title is more complicated than the recipe!

If you don't happen to have Madeleine tins in

your inventory, you can improvise. But according to Frances, the real thing is inexpensive and readily available at cookware stores.

PETITES MADELEINES CORDON BLEU

4 large eggs
1¹/₂ cups sugar
1¹/₄ cups butter, melted
2¹/₃ cups cake flour
1 tablespoon lemon juice

Beat eggs until light. Add sugar and melted butter, beating until smooth. Add flour and lemon juice, and stir until well blended. Pour into well-buttered Madeleine tins and bake at 325 degrees for 25 minutes.

Another friend gets extra credit for her imaginative idea: hard-boiled eggs, each with a silly face drawn on the shell with Magic Marker, brought in a basket. And no, she never forgets the little packets of salt. Maybe eggs are not teatime tidbits, but if they don't get eaten for lunches, they can eventually, like flowers, get thrown out. It doesn't matter— they're for fun.

Anyway, the gist of the tea-for-two idea (or coffee, or juice) is that the food is really just background for your visit, a way to move the four walls back a little—and if your patient only manages a sip and a bite, well, the pleasant feeling is still there.

If you did a quick survey down a hospital corridor, I think you'd find that the one food treat that sounds the most appealing to the most patients is ice cream and its variations: sherbert, frozen yogurt, a milkshake. Obviously you'd have to run at the speed of light to get an ice cream cone to your patient in halfway decent shape, but you can pull off a milkshake by using the fruit salad trick: freeze it first so that it arrives at the hospital icy cold. If you can manage this, you'll get raves.

When you can't stay for the cleanup, or if you're sending food via courier, try to stick with non-messy non-perishables, like a tin of hard candies, assorted Lifesaver packs, even lollipops (all are a quick antidote to "medicine mouth"). A bowl of slivered almonds (unsalted) mixed with white seedless raisins makes wonderful munching, and the combination also happens to be tops in nutritional value. Or put together a "survival kit" of small packets that can be tucked into a bedside drawer for midnight-hunger emergencies.

If a family member is staying late or overnight, you can be a help by fixing a sandwich, a juice, and a brownie "for Joe." Remembering Joe and sparing him the vending machine blues will mean as much to your patient as anything you could do for her.

Betty and Harry stopped by the hospital one evening when they knew I was "sleeping over." They brought a sturdy box packed with wonderful midnight food just for *ME*. Oh, I do remember how good that food tasted. But even more vividly, I remember how Lee's eyes lighted up . . . when I had assumed they would never again remember how to. The loving couple did no more than step to the door and say goodnight, but their gift defies description.

You might remember just such a gift for a night when the only prognosis is zero. The family person who is there would snort if you asked, "May I get you something to eat?" But that box, with everything wrapped so carefully . . . well, I even remember exactly how the paper napkin was folded into a swan.

Special Food for Special Patients

When your patient is back home and on a limited diet, you can help relieve the boredom of bland food with your own versions of old standbys— *comfort foods*—that the patient's family may not have time to prepare. Here's where the flair becomes a real challenge, as you come up with ways to dress the simplest of foods in gourmet disguise.

Applesauce, for instance, can be applesauce . . . or it can be Dorothy's version: smooth as double-backed satin, chilled, with a sprinkle of cinnamon on top.

DOROTHY'S APPLESAUCE

Use tart, firm apples such as Winesap, Rome Beauty, Courtland, Stayman, or Baldwin. Wash the apples, cut into quarters, and core, but don't peel them. The peelings add to flavor in cooking.

Simmer in a little water until soft. Then process in a food processor. If you prefer a coarser applesauce, simply continue cooking until the apples disintegrate, and remove the pieces of peel with a fork or tongs. Transfer to a bowl and add fresh lemon juice and honey to taste. Sprinkle with cinnamon just before serving or delivering.

The cook responsible for this delicacy has not given quantities, as you can see. I guess you know that great cooks are often like that.

My mother, for instance, trying to tell me how to duplicate her biscuits said, quite seriously, "If the milk is sour, you use more soda."

I got nowhere with "More soda than what?"

But some of you, I bet, will know exactly what she meant.

My own favorite "special food," baked custard from the simplest mixture I know about, is a can't-fail recipe (though I did wreck one batch by putting curry on top instead of nutmeg, but it *was* midnight). Different ages, tastes, degrees of misery — all patients love its slick feel and taste, warm or cold. Most baked custards refuse to guarantee that they'll be smooooooth clear to the bottom, right? There's that watery stuff that appears too often and then the cook mutters, "I guess the oven was . . ." or "Maybe the eggs were . . ." But this recipe, with all its 3's, is always cooperative, clear to the bottom of every cup.

JANE'S BAKED CUSTARD

> *3 slightly beaten eggs*
> *3 tablespoons sugar*
>   *Dash salt, optional*
> *3 cups scalded milk*
> *1 teaspoon vanilla*
>   *Nutmeg*

Combine eggs, sugar, and salt. Slowly add milk and vanilla. Pour into 6 to 8 custard cups and sprinkle with nutmeg. Place in a shallow pan filled with an inch of hot tap water and bake at 350 degrees for about an hour, until a knife comes out clean.

Remember bread pudding? I'd always confused it with milktoast and never much cared for the idea, until Bertha brought some during an illness and re-minded me that this is a different breed altogether. Surprise! It's so tasty that your youngsters will gobble up the leftovers.

BERTHA'S BREAD PUDDING

$2^1/_4$ cups milk, scalded
2 slightly beaten eggs
2 cups buttered bread cubes
$^1/_2$ cup brown sugar
1 teaspoon vanilla
$^1/_2$ teaspoon nutmeg
$^1/_2$ teaspoon cinnamon
$^1/_4$ teaspoon salt, optional
$^1/_2$ cup seedless raisins

Slowly combine milk and eggs. Pour over bread cubes. Stir in remaining ingredients, and pour into a greased 8-inch round baking dish. Place in a shallow pan filled with an inch of hot tap water and bake at 350 degrees for 45 minutes or until firm. Serve with cream or thin (pourable) custard.

If you have time to make a soup from scratch, you can plant a star on your crown, or at least think one is there. Nothing else combines freshness, ease of swallowing, nutrition, and taste so perfectly, *and* provides vertical storage. Whoa . . . vertical what?

It doesn't sound flair-ish, but it is (literally) the height of thoughtful packaging. If you'll deliver your soup in a Mason jar or pitcher with a lid, it can keep for days without taking up much refrigerator space, and it can be stored and poured from the same container. That, I call handy.

Here's a basic vegetable soup that friends of mine have nourished our family with.

VEGETABLE SOUP

> 2 *quarts cold water*
> 3 *to 4 pounds beef soup bone*
> 1 *small onion, quartered*
> 1 *teaspoon salt, optional*
> 2 *cups tomatoes*
> 2 *cups green beans*
> 1 *cup diced potato*
> *1/2 cup chopped celery*
> *1/4 cup rice or barley*
> *1/4 cup chopped cabbage*
> 5 *or 6 carrots, sliced*
> 6 *sprigs parsley*

Cook bone, onion, and salt in the water for 2 hours. Add remaining vegetables and cook 1 hour longer. (You can substitute chicken stock for the soup bone and water.)

A truly wonderful soup that takes a little more finesse is this Fresh Cauliflower Soup from a mother's kitchen to me and my family after a hospital bout.

FRESH CAULIFLOWER SOUP

6 tablespoons butter or margarine, divided
1/2 cup chopped onion
1 cup chopped celery
1 carrot, chopped
1 head cauliflower, in flowerets
1 tablespoon chopped parsley
8 cups chicken broth
1 teaspoon dried leaf tarragon
1/2 teaspoon whole peppercorns
1/2 bay leaf
2/3 cup flour
2 cups milk
1 cup half-and-half
Salt, if desired

In a large saucepan melt 2 tablespoons butter. Saute onions until transparent. Add celery and carrot, and cook 2 minutes. Add cauliflower and parsley. Cover. Simmer 15 minutes. Add chicken broth.

Make a bouquet garni by wrapping tarragon, peppercorns, and bay leaf in a small piece of cheesecloth.

Secure with string, and add to saucepan. Bring soup to boil, then reduce heat and simmer 5 minutes.

Melt remaining 4 tablespoons butter in a 2-quart saucepan. Stir in flour and cook 1 minute. Remove from heat. Gradually stir in milk. Return to heat and bring to a boil, stirring constantly until mixture thickens. Stir in half-and-half.

Add milk mixture to soup. Salt to taste. Simmer 20 minutes. Discard bouquet garni. Puree soup, if you wish.

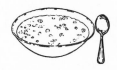

When you don't have time to chop, dice, or wrap peppercorns, and you don't have hours to supervise your stove, you can get almost as much credit (at least at my house) for this next recipe. Not only does it take no time; it takes no stove.

Lee's sister, here from North Carolina during Lee's illness, was so taken by its delicious taste when Jean, the "cook," brought it over that she copied the recipe and tried it on a group of her super-cook friends back home. According to her report, the Fruit Plus, for all its simplicity, was a hurrah-success, even outside a sickroom.

For your patient-friends, it has the added quality of going down as easily as Jello, and it has a lot more texture.

JEAN'S FRUIT PLUS

- 1 lg. can chunk or crushed pineapple, with juice
- 2 cans mandarin oranges, with juice of 1 can (discard juice of 2nd can)
- 1 small jar maraschino cherries, drained
- 1 small package vanilla instant pudding
- 3 or 4 bananas

Combine first 4 ingredients and let stand 6 to 8 hours in the refrigerator. Slice bananas and add just before delivering.

When food is going to a truly ill patient, who *must* have sustenance, we should pull out the stops to make what we offer as appealing as possible.

I've known a few people who would swallow pureed mush of Anything without squawking, but most of them were under two. Most very weak patients really do try — doctor's orders — but they feel force-fed much of the time.

When a friend shows up with something different, something pretty and palatable, it's great to watch the return of a spark of anticipation, to see your patient be actually tempted. So do use all the tricks up your sleeve: the twist of lemon peel, the shaved bit of semi-sweet chocolate, the cinnamon stick, the icing design— go for it!

Food for the Family

Late one evening after an especially long day at the hospital, unwilling to face one more piece of pizza or limp lump of meat-in-bun in a greasy wrapper, I yanked open my refrigerator door, determined to mine its depths for something, *anything,* from a food group other than "fast."

My prayers were answered: my friend Joan had beaten me to the punch! I've no recollection of how she got into the house, but the results of her ingenuity were as bright as a flash bulb in the dark.

Right then and there, at the age of who's counting, I had my first truly great experience with raw vegetables. Joan had filled a clear bowl with chipped ice and a squeeze of lemon, and this became the base for long slivers of scraped carrot, de-stringed celery, sliced cucumber, and chunks of cauliflower and broccoli. Ah, what a delight to bite into something that actually crunched back!

I continue to feel slight surprise that plain old raw vegetables can score so high on the scale of great food. Never, though, has the combination tasted as fresh and crisp as when my mouth and spirits were dull and cottony from hospital detail. And you wonder what you can do for a dear friend who's where I was?

Now I'm a convert. I regularly fix a similar mixture, and children know they can *always* reach into it without permission. The addition of ranch dressing as a dip makes it a perfect lunch.

Another of my best remembered friend-dishes during family illness was Sydel's meat loaf. I'm not including the recipe itself since she insists it's quite standard. It was delicious, and I hope yours is, too. What made her flair special was that, since I was the sole recipient, she brought the loaf already subdivided into separate packets for freezing, the stack topped with a container of superb tomato sauce. For me, meat loaf was a perfect choice because I could eat it hot, cold, or in-between, and even in sandwiches. Each way, and each time I unfroze a packet, I had a different meal.

Elisabeth doubtless hit a record in generosity by arriving with an entire platter of beef tenderloins nudged with fresh parsley. And fresh asparagus. *And* honest Hollandaise sauce, not the ersatz kind. Now, if I were to dare put butter and lemon in the same room together, they'd run to opposite corners, so real Hollandaise is a treat for me on a par with rarities like caviar. And there I was with enough gorgeous meat to feed an army. With judicious wrapping and freezing, I had filet mignon for months, and she claimed it was just the leftovers from her family's Sunday roast. Some leftovers!

Even if your refrigerator yields up humbler remains from last night's dinner, this is still a perfect way to help out a solitary caregiver who has no use for an entire casserole.

The two categories of full meal foods that rate highest with my pool of experts on Culinary Rescue are chicken dishes and salads. Both of these take well to travel and to minor abuse, like not being eaten hot, or right away, or all at once (or with a fork). Laila's unusual chicken salad combines the best of both.

LAILA'S CHICKEN SALAD

   $1/2$ cup sour cream
   $1/4$ cup mayonnaise
   $1/2$ teaspoon salt
   2 cups diced cooked chicken
   $1/2$ cup toasted slivered almonds
   $1/2$ cup diced celery
      Lettuce
   1 can (1 lb.) dark red cherries, optional

Blend sour cream, mayonnaise, and salt. Add chicken, nuts, and celery. Toss and chill. Serve on lettuce bed. For pizzazz, drain and chill cherries and add carefully just before serving.

Most people like pasta salads. They keep especially well, make good nibble-food, and go with anything that someone else might bring. We enjoyed Gertrude's success with this one.

GERTRUDE'S ZESTY PASTA SALAD

- $^1/_2$ cup mayonnaise
- $^1/_3$ cup grated parmesan cheese
- 2 tablespoons milk
- $1^1/_2$ cups smoked meat, cubed
- 1 cup chopped green pepper
- 1 cup cherry tomato halves
- 1 cup (4 oz.) shell macaroni, cooked and drained
- $^1/_4$ cup chopped onion
  Salt, if desired

Combine mayonnaise, parmesan cheese, and milk. Mix well, then gently mix in the remaining ingredients. Salt to taste. Chill several hours.

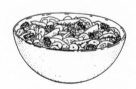

Every one of my friends has a favorite chicken dish in her arsenal of Food for Families, but I've chosen this one because even now, twelve years after it was delivered to my door by a friend who *walked* two miles to bring it, I can still call up its tangy, tender taste and the dinner-party flair of its looks.

CAROL'S CHICKEN BREAST SUPREME

4 whole chicken breasts, skin removed
2 teaspoons salt
1 teaspoon pepper
6 tablespoons butter, divided
1/2 cup white wine
1/3 cup chopped onion
1 cup sour cream
1/4 cup sliced ripe olives
1/4 cup chopped chives

Season chicken breasts with salt and pepper. Saute in 4 tablespoons butter until golden. Pour wine over chicken, cover, and simmer until tender (about 30 minutes). Remove chicken and place in serving dish.

Remove liquid from skillet and reserve. Add remaining 2 tablespoons butter to the skillet and saute onions until tender. Stir in sour cream, olives, and reserved liquid. Heat but do not boil. Pour over chicken and garnish with chives.

If the mouths that you're filling include a number of small ones, you could try your own version of an idea that has always pleased the children in my life down to the tips of their toes. Its success comes, I'm sure, from any child's delight in knowing he has something all-to-himself, especially when times aren't easy.

Fill a picnic basket with separate sacks for each child (names on them, of course), and a bright tablecloth, napkins, cups —everything needed for the children to fix their own table, outdoors if possible. Into each sack, none quite the same, pack four or five individually wrapped foods to make a meal, for example: fried chicken, cherry tomatoes, carrot sticks, celery spread with cream cheese, a cupcake, a drink, and a surprise trinket at the bottom.

Children love unwrapping their riches and laying out the party, and how they need an entertaining time-out from having to behave like little adults when there's an upset in their lives.

These ideas are just a few from the many that my friends have used over the years to see me and others through the day-to-day food demands that take a back seat to illness. They certainly don't cover the cooking front. They're more like teasers, to remind you of favorites of your own or to give you a chance to try something different. And to remind you that food is more than a special gift: it's crucial.

Without my friends' efforts I wouldn't have pitifully starved to death. I would have lived on exactly what other families of seriously ill patients live on: as little as necessary, whatever's handy and quick, nutrition no concern and since money always is, the cheaper the better.

Coffee and donuts.

Ask anybody weathering a crisis a food-related question, as in "Can I get you something to eat?" and you'll get a distracted response that manages "no," or "yes," with equal enthusiasm. But then place a large helping of your home-cooked specialty in front of that same friend and you'll watch it disappear in seconds. (I once saw the husband of a hospitalized friend go through the better part of a pot roast and then ask blankly, "More what?" when seconds were offered.)

When something is pressing at your very center, you forget that part of the ache may be hunger. And nobody can run on empty or low-octane forever. I know for a fact that friends' cooking has saved me from patienthood myself more than once. And I know for a fact that *thank you* — as in thanksgiving, as in "let us give thanks" — is never more heartfelt than when it is said over food.

chapter seven

Troubled Waters

MOST OF US have no trouble expressing our sympathy when an illness or accident strikes someone near. WHY, then, is it so difficult for us to walk up to a friend and say "I'm sorry to hear about your son's trouble . . . your house . . . your miscarriage . . . your divorce."

Because I'm embarrassed.

Because I feel helpless.

Because someone might think it was an intrusion.

Because "sorry" doesn't MEAN enough. Geez, you can be "sorry" you stepped on someone's waxed linoleum before it was dry.

That's a sampling of the reaction I got from early morning fellow-walkers in Loose Park when I conducted my informal survey. I wasn't looking for scientific answers from experts in sociology and psychology; I wanted opinions from everyday people. And did I get them!

No one knew the purpose of my questions; no one really knew *me* except as someone they pass regularly on the two-mile path around the park. The little dogs that walk with me are such an endearing opening act that I had the perfect casual setting for the variety of frank answers I hoped I'd get.

But I got more than that. I got explosiveness! It was like pulling a plug: the swirl of response seemed to have been dammed up, waiting for a chance to spill. I couldn't have asked for better evidence that we have a widely-shared problem.

Nobody said, "Come on, who says it's difficult?"

Everyone agreed that we, as friends, feel awkward and unsure about managing the Being Sorry that's our part of another's bad times. Everyone had experienced the problem in some form, and everyone had an opinion.

Some Reasons We Have Difficulty

If your mind is whirring with possible answers to the "why," so is mine. As with most answers to difficult questions, this one seems to be a combination of a lot of partial "becauses." And all of those reasons add up to one that takes us right to the heart of our individuality as people:

"It's so hard to *KNOW*."

Up until now, we've been talking mostly about illness, where the pain is identifiable, where we have a measurable situation against which to gauge the probable value of our ways of helping. But when a friend's misfortune strikes heart and soul more than body— as with divorce, bankruptcy, legal problems, a teenager in trouble, the loss of a job or a home— the situation is not nearly so well-defined. You can't always have an insight to the emotions churning underneath, and it's harder to know just how to put your wanting to help into action.

What If I Say the Wrong Thing?

There's a two-sided scenario that plays itself inside my head (more of a nightmare, really) that goes like this:

I run into a friend, Margaret, the week after she's auctioned her houseful of heirloom furniture to pay off business debts. I tell her how sorry I am, that I know how very much her grandmother's antiques meant to her. The next morning (this is a nightmare, remember, so it doesn't have to be logical) I open the newspaper and there is her letter:

Dear Abby:

    We've recently lost nearly everything because of the failure of our business. I'm trying so hard to keep my head held up and get back to normal, but my friends won't stop reminding me of our misfortune. Just yesterday one of these busybodies walked right up to me in the market and made a great big deal out of it! Please let people know that the last thing I need is their pity.

Then the flip-side of the nightmare:

This time, instead of offering Margaret my sympathy I had settled for greeting her casually. So she mails off this letter:

Dear Abby:

    We've recently lost just about everything because of the failure of our business — including, it seems, our friends. Yesterday I ran into one of them in the market and she barely even spoke to me. Please let people know that anything can be endured as long as friends stick by you and don't act as if that "anything" is taboo.

If Margaret's husband had suffered a stroke instead of financial collapse, she would not feel defensive at all. But when pride is involved, and hurt, a sense of defeat, a threat to self-esteem — that's where we run up against the damned-if-you-do-damned-if-you-don't kind of quandary from which mind-boggles are made. We can't know when our well-meant words and gestures might produce pain instead of comfort in a troubled situation. But — and this is a very large *BUT* — we do know that saying and doing nothing simply doesn't advance us one inch in our desire to give support. In the results of my straw poll, most people agreed that they'd rather be blamed for doing than for not doing.

Five Suggestions

The problem is always going to be there. Our best bet is to live with it and to give our best effort at comfort and help. Assuming that we share that basic thought, I'll forge ahead with five suggestions.

1.

If you're going to speak your sorry-ness, keep your statement simple and then keep going.

To drop "I'm sorry about Tim's trouble . . . ." and then wait for the friend you've intercepted to take over is poor indeed. What can she say? "Me, too?" "Thank you?" And then what? Hearts have a way of swelling up into throats, and you may both stand there helplessly sparring with Enormity. If you want to be good at simply speaking the words straight out, you need to be willing to take the weight of the awkwardness onto yourself.

I'm sorry about _____. That's a rough

*one, I know, but maybe it'll help a little if you'll
let me _____ on next Tuesday.
I'll check on Monday. Meantime, how about
a cup of coffee right now?*

*I'm sorry about _____. I know
there's just never a way to make those words
say enough, but I had to try because you've been
so much in my thoughts. Would a
dinner invitation for next Monday make any
sense? I'll be in touch Monday morning.*

*"I'm sorry about _____.
I hope you know how well you're doing at
handling it. I give you lots of credit, and
you should too. Would you want to come by
tomorrow or Thursday after we get through
work . . . and just talk? Or just sit on the porch
with a dog beside you for patting?
No food, drink, or advice?"*

Your goal is to get to the point where you can
handle "I'm sorry" in such a way that the friend
you've spoken to doesn't *have* to talk about IT at all,
but can just respond to the much simpler business
of coffee, or whatever.

Rehearse. (Don't laugh. Rehearsal does help.)
Work out ahead of time your own ways to go on after saying "I'm sorry about . . ." instead of leaving a
hole. Knowing what you're going to say will give you

confidence, and you won't have any problem supervising your voice and directing your eyes straight at your friend's.

2.

Show how you feel by putting your arms around your troubled friend.

This is no time for diffident cheek-pecking or waiting to see what the other will do. A loving hug is the kind of warming statement that needs no words. Enfold! And be grateful that we human beings still have such a powerful antidote to misery.

3.

Beware of gossip.

Personal misfortunes, unlike illness or injury, bring about a whole web of unverified rumor, half-truths, and innuendos.

Here, instead of a straightforward call from a relative to say that "Betsy went into St. Paul's this afternoon for surgery," news of Betsy's losing her job often gets to friends and co-workers second-hand, around the water fountain or at Friday night's cocktail party. The "news" grows with each retelling. Everybody wants to know the whole story, and since they don't get it, they let their imaginations fill the gaps. "I heard she was drinking on the job." "I heard it was drugs."

Please, as a real helper, avoid discussing with

others your troubled friend's situation. Settle for not knowing the details, and put all your concern instead into that direct "I'm sorry about _____" contact with your friend. If your coffee invitation does happen to result in shared confidences, then do your friend the added kindness of turning aside others' inquiries to you.

4.

Be prepared for failure.

A gifted young pianist friend of mind avoids terror before a monstrously difficult section in her concert performances by "practicing for the worst that could happen: total panic, a sudden blank." She says, "I practice failure, and I can make it *very* real." You should do the same. Go ahead and assume that your friend will respond brusquely. It can happen.

You: I want to tell you how sorry I am about

_____ .

She: I don't want to talk about it!

You: Can I _____?
He: No, there's nothing anyone can do.

Then what?
Then you have to hang on hard to the fact that this person you're trying to help gets special treat-

ment. You can't turn on your heel with a red face and a muttered, "Have it your way, then." You need instead to get both of you onto other, safer ground. It's not easy, but if you've thought ahead maybe you'll be able to stay afloat.

I can see how you'd feel ....

Or, without a shadow of a huff:

That's fine, Mary dear. I'll be in touch.

5.

And do be in touch, whatever the response to "I'm sorry."

Down the days from now, when too many friends drift away, figuring the "worst is over," your reminders that you haven't forgotten can be a big, big help. The "worst" can be a long, lonely road.

Stay With It

A friend of mine had an accident quite a while ago. It was completely unavoidable: a little girl on a bicycle swerved suddenly off the sidewalk and in front of his car. My friend, a driver with a perfect record, hit his brakes but couldn't avoid running into her. The child died.

Steve (I don't want to use his real name) was understandably devastated for a long, long time. I know he'll never truly recover, in the sense of getting "over" it. But his sanity and self-esteem were saved, I think, because of the actions of friends, one in particular, who saw through Steve's insistence that he was "perfectly fine."

Will checked in with Steve weekly after "the worst" was over. He didn't pry or give advice or wax philosophic; he just stopped by with a new novel to lend, or to watch a ball game on TV, or to get advice on fixing a pesky sprinkler system. It was Will who noticed when Steve started going into a tailspin—drinking too much, eating poorly, letting his apartment go to pieces. It was Will who checked around and got the name of a highly recommended psychiatrist from another friend, and who called the doctor to ask if he could see Steve.

And it was Will who sat down with Steve and said, "My friend, I know what you're going through, and I don't know how you've managed this far without help. Please, would you do this: would you talk to Joe Darien on Wednesday evening?"

Today Steve would tell you that Dr. Darien saved his life. I don't know if he credits Will or not, but *I* surely do. Everyone else moved on, subscribing to Steve's apparent vote to consider the accident "over and done." Will created his own great definition for "keeping in touch."

It's true that we can't always know how others feel in such situations. It's also true that they themselves often don't know, and can't see ahead to the next step, or the next after that. However beautifully a friend seems to be adjusting, we can be sure that deep hurts don't mysteriously metabolize into run-of-the-mill setbacks. They don't just go away after a good night's sleep or a few days' rest. It takes a special kind of friend to be patient enough — thoughtful enough — to hang in there and to keep remembering, with thoughtful invitations, spontaneous calls, small gifts that say *This made me think of you.*

What About Gifts?

Of course, you could do many of the job-gifts or take many of the wrapped ones discussed in earlier chapters, or you could simmer up a pot of vegetable soup for quart jars of delivered nourishment, same as before. But I think you'll continue to feel as though you're clapping with one hand.

When a friend is having a rough time, ordinary responsiveness to *things* is understandably limited. Things are just . . . things; they don't register. The kinds of gifts that work here aren't practical, they're ones that say something about your friendship and take note of the specialness of your friend.

Don't worry, I'm not going to tell you your gift must be Meaningful to make any impression. I'm just talking about making a connection between the gift and the person.

Let's say that you're thinking of Jennifer plodding through an unhappy time in her life, and you'd love to give her an unexpected something to pick up her spirits.

Like what?

Well, focus your thinking right now on Jennifer the person. Where and how does she stand out in your memory?

Go ahead and write down a list of words or phrases that add up to what you know of Jennifer. Try to think of clues from the tennis games or business meetings or dinner parties or exercise classes you've shared. Move her around in your mind into all different situations, wherever you've been near enough to each other for you to have had a chance to notice or hear a possible answer to what you need now.

Keep going until you have a smattering that might look a bit like this:

-- loves mysteries

-- cantaloupe

-- no green

-- roses

-- early riser

-- country western music

-- supports zoo

144

If you look at your listing in a couple of weeks, you might join Robert Browning in his admission, when asked about the meaning of a particular line of his poem, "When I wrote that, God and I knew what I meant; now only God knows." Never mind, nobody's going to see your list and think you've been out in the sun too long.

If you're older than Jennifer and have known her since she was a bitsy, let some reminiscing get into your list: your remembering her persistent requests for new boxes of crayons when she was eight just might warm her worn-out self as she reads your note that says her Crayola hankering from childhood made you choose this small framed Degas print for her bedroom.

Now I don't know this Jennifer, but from that list above I might suggest you choose a cassette tape of Alabama, the great C and W group. You could say on your card: "This says Jennifer-music to me and it's wrapped with a blue ribbon because that's what you deserve."

Jennifer would know you'd been thinking of her — *HER* — in a way that a potted plant or perfume or candy, nice as they are, couldn't show. Incidentally, some variation of this list method will come in handy for any gift-giving. It's fun, like a puzzle, and when the tumblers fall together in the right combination, you can practically taste the satisfaction.

You may be thinking that this doesn't seem like much, that the added "fit" in the choice of a gift or the words on a card is a small gesture. Small, but mighty. It's a reminder of your *noticing*. It may not mend a marriage or broken dreams, but I think it can go a good way toward shoring up a shaken Self.

Knowing your friend, you will be able to find other ways to keep the continuity of your concern going, without poking incessantly at the wound. Nobody but a chronic complainer appreciates being asked over and over, "Are you sure you're doing all right?" And that question is a woefully inadequate one when you already know the answer can't possibly be an unqualified yes. What's needed is the reassurance that your friendship is there, strong as ever, whatever the problem at hand.

If you've done the mental exercise to come up with a gift-match, then you've already thought through the ways that your life and your friend's intersect. Now you can plant that reference firmly in mind — or top drawer — to make sure you don't miss any opportunities for connecting.

Yes, of course your friend will know you're going out of your way when you call to make sure that she doesn't miss the special on Agatha Christie, or when you send a copy of an article on a new hybrid rose that caught your eye.

She'll know, and it's the knowing that will strengthen her. The Simon and Garfunkel song, "Bridge over Troubled Waters" is a beautiful metaphor, but that bridge doesn't build overnight or with one grand, selfless gesture. It builds when you keep at it.

That doesn't mean there's no place for grand gestures.

Holding a Fundraiser

What about giving help in a situation that involves material loss, such as a fire, flood, or burglary, or when insurance doesn't cover an expensive operation or extended care? What about those hardships that leave a friend or neighbor with a crushing financial burden?

Obviously, you're not one to partake in hand-wringing with the Milling-Around Inadequates, nor are you the type who can "leave it lie" and watch the chips fall through your binoculars. You want to do something significant to help the family rebuild.

Well, take a deep breath.

Beyond the large number of minor ways to lend a hand, what's really called for when there's serious financial hardship is Help with a capital H. My capital H advice is that you roll up your sleeves, brush up on your organization skills and plan a fundraising event. Even if you've never done this sort of thing before, you may surprise yourself. All it takes, I promise, is energy and *wanting* to.

Here's how to go about it:

First, establish a fund by opening an account at your local bank. This is free, and it will help you and your stricken friend keep track of donations.

Next, sit down and make two lists, first of the

circle of friends you think will want to help; then of the more casual friends, acquaintances and coworkers you'll want to notify or invite.

Now you'll need to come up with a type of event — or several to choose from — to fit the skills and interests of the inner circle of people you plan to approach for help.

A word of warning here. You and others are going to put a good amount of time and energy into this undertaking, so you should weigh carefully the profit potential of the various events available to you. A bake sale, for example, might not bring in enough to be worth marshaling all those resources, unless it's spread over several days and is done on a major scale. You'll have to do some hard figuring.

There are many, many possible fundraisers to choose from, including, to name just a few:

-- a car wash (great if teen labor is available)

-- a Walk-A-Thon (supporters "back" participants by pledging so much per mile)

-- a rummage sale

-- a pancake breakfast

Many successful events are combinations: a raffle, for example, can easily be added to any of the above suggestions.

One of the best benefits I've ever seen (and a

big money-maker) was an "Unusual Auction." People donated anything they could think of, from artwork to homemade preserves, from myself-as-a-slave to a catered dinner for two.

Some ideas seem to work better in some communities than others, and you may want to check with local non-profit groups for tips. If you have a friend in Lions Club or know a PTA mother, that would be a good place to start.

Then, if you haven't already managed the necessary conference, you should sit down with the family you're trying to help and, with your enthusiasm and energy at the fore, explain your great idea and make sure you have their blessing. If there are children in the family, enlist their help. Give each child, each family member, a place in the sun.

And be sure to get the names of every group and organization each family member belongs to, so that you can add the names on those rosters to the list of contacts you've already started.

And now . . . get on the phone.

"Whew," you're saying. "This is a BIG project." Yes it is, and it is definitely not for everybody. But you may be surprised once you get the ball rolling to find yourself charged up and actually enjoying it. You'll also find that where supporting a good cause close to home is concerned, friends will rally around and volunteer their help. You'll get good at delegating, fast.

I suggest you find several people right at the start who are willing to take on organizing one aspect of your benefit, such as

> -- arranging publicity,
>
> -- finding a location,
>
> -- enlisting workers,
>
> -- soliciting donations,
>
> -- printing tickets.

Make your own primary job running the command post and coordinating the committees.

Try to treat the project like a job. Allocate a specific work period for it each day, and keep a notebook for all your checklists. Use a calendar-timetable for the different parts of the job:

> 3/19: Sue contact Daylight Donuts
>
> Lucille confirm Lions' Club available
>
> Bobby's class put up posters at school

Then, on 3/20, you check with Sue, Lucille and Bobby for reports. Keep careful accounting of out-of-pocket expenses so they can be reimbursed. And try to keep track of your own time; later it may be useful to you and others to know the hours involved.

One final point (important!): be sure, when you're enlisting volunteers, to remember that you'll need help afterwards for

     -- clean-up,

     -- handling unsold items,

     -- taking down posters,

     -- sacking trash.

A friend of mine found out the hard way that all such jobs have to be anticipated. She was still "winding up" her fundraiser all by herself a week later. Trash and leftovers don't simply disappear!

Once your big project has gone off without a hitch, let the family you're helping know who they may thank and for what. If you have energy left, your finale could be an offer to help with notes.

This isn't intended as a primer on fundraising, but it should give you an idea that heading up such an event doesn't take particular skills or even contacts.

If you do decide to take on this Big Job as

your gift, you'll be giving much more than money. And who knows, maybe afterwards you'll write that primer for others.

chapter eight

After a Death

YOU'VE ALREADY FOUND that all answers to "If there's anything I can do" start with being thoughtful. It's thoughtfulness that gets you "inside the skin" of the friend you want to help so that you can find the right responses to fit that particular friend.

After a death, you will redouble every earlier effort at inside-the-skin thoughtfulness, feeling *with* your friend in grief.

You'll find that you already have a good start. Your built-up store of ways to give personal, practical help; your comfort level with difficult visits; your shored-up determination to follow through with ongoing reminders of your love . . . all these will give you ballast and confidence in yourself now, in this bleakest of bad times. But there is one switch — a big one. After a death, if you're truly to give help, you need to have spent part of your thoughtfulness on yourself.

Why? Because I honestly believe you can't do much for the friend who needs your help in the overwhelming pain suffered because of a death, until you have first worked out your own answers to all the immediate external demands that follow a death.

All too often, in my experience, people meet each new death among friends and relatives with the same inner tussles:

What shall I do?

Should I go to the house?

Should I send flowers?

Is the mortuary a must?

Need I go to an out-of-town funeral?

Must I wear black?

Should I pay a visit?

Shall I take the children?

We get so tangled in the "mechanics" that surround us after a death that we're not free to help as our best selves. The fact is, the deciding almost *has* to be done before the need for action comes up. Time is a real consideration after a death.

With all the other physical, mental and emotional battles being fought by good friends, you have time on your side when you want to help. You can plan, discard, wait until you have an open afternoon.

You can make mistakes of judgment and then go back and rectify them a bit later.

After a death, you can't. *After* a death is for all the future as far as your friend is concerned, but for you Time becomes a tyrant.

The important thing is to make those choices — on flowers, notes, funeral attire and attendance, cross-country travel — and then stand by them. Otherwise, we'll go on with the waffling indecision that gets in our way each time we most want to be strong and resourceful. Now, ahead of time, without the pressure for immediate action, watch and listen and adapt from your present experiences.

Pay attention especially to the more thoughtfully enacted alternatives to established tradition . . . like this great variation:

The fine man whose large funeral was a tribute to his high standing in our community had always loved a good band. He had no affinity for orchestras, but a band . . . now *that* was music!

After the formal seating, after the family members, the minister and the altar attendants had taken their places, from the foyer of this enormous church came the loud and heart-lifting measures of "The Saints Go Marching In," with every piece of band equipment thoroughly engaged in filling the massive space. No muted trumpet or half-blown trombone! No death-roll from the drum! Full and glorious, the sounds marched down the center aisle to the altar.

Though no doubt there were those who rolled their eyes in objection, I think I was not the only one who half-expected to hear the man they honored call out in the voice we'd all known in its joyous resonance, "Great! Keep Going!"

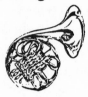

Making Choices

No, I'm not suggesting that you must chuck any of your old ideas because they won't do anymore. Actually I love the familiar church rituals, in part because they *are* so familiar and so much a part of my past. I'm simply saying that it's good to be free, after a death, to honor love and not necessarily litany. And I'm saying that the best responses come from a calm, inside sureness of knowing our actions are personal and true.

We learn from each other. A friend of mine taught me in a startling way the value of sorting out the answers to "What should I do?" by starting from "What is right for *me*?"

Linda, a former classmate and close friend, lost her husband to a heart attack. The funeral was on a

cold, rainy, late afternoon, as they always seem to me
to be, whatever the season. By the time the services
were over it was dark. Those of us who were close
enough to Linda to gather at her home afterward
followed Linda's car through the dreary, slippery
streets deeply wishing (I know I was) that there were
some way to spare her this first coming home to a
cold, dark, empty house. We all straggled damply
through the front door to find . . . lights on, fire-
place acrackle, fresh coffee and sandwich makings
laid out on the dining table.

Grace stepped out of the kitchen with her apron
on.

"I know I'm early, dear," she said to Linda, "But
I wanted to save you the hostessing."

The lift of Linda's shoulders and the gratitude
in her voice when she said, "This is lovely," couldn't
have been staged. I found Grace alone later and told
her I thought her "house-warming" was the single
most thoughtful act I had ever seen.

"I don't go to funerals, you see," she said, without a hint of righteousness or apology. "So I thought
I could help by doing this instead."

What a satisfactory approach! How much better than the hand-wringing of the acquaintance I
ran into later that week, who babbled on miserably

about how "I should have gone...but the weather...
and I just hate...I hope Linda understands...."

Grace's calm aside, I realize that what each
person decides to do after getting notice of a death
is never going to be a complete and easy matter,
solved by the making of a list. Stepping in to warm
a house, for instance, might never "work" for a single other person.

I have learned, though, that thinking out atti-
tudes and actions ahead of time can make a big difference in turning a whirlpool of uncertainty into a
manageable ripple. Having a straight line to follow
is a very big help. And thinking ahead now about
how you want to manage your participation in the
"mechanics" that follow a death, hard as it seems, is
much easier than scrambling questions and answers
on the day you need them.

Talking with Friends

It isn't necessary, though, to think inside an
isolation booth. Don't you normally sound out your
friends for opinions on how they will act in almost
any situation, from nuisance calls to social introduc-
tions to an all-out nuclear war? With almost every
topic that holds sway over our lives, we try out our
ideas, pool our resources, compare and contrast the
opinions of our peers — that's how we help settle
our own.

Yet most of us have no clear idea of how we

will handle ourselves after a death. I think it is be-cause — let's face it — we're scared to death to talk about Death. That reticence must be spooned into us with our Gerber's because it is pandemic: the subject of death is a conversation inhibitor with no equal.

Yet I think if we set out to talk about death, we could get rid of some of the shrouds and mental cobwebs, at least with regard to what friends can and/or should do.

I can picture you, having chosen a good time, asking a good friend, "Let me bounce this off the wall . . ." or "Let me get your reaction to this . . ." and following up with one of the questions that churn in your mind when you try to chart your course af-ter news of a death.

What do you think about friends expecting to come by the house after a funeral . . . expecting almost a party? Is it hard on the family or do you think it's a good idea? Should friends wait to be asked?

Or

What would you think about going to a funeral without going to the internment? Would you need to make an excuse?"

I can even imagine a time that would be right

for tackling this stickler:

> *John, you're an expert at handling*
> *difficult questions in your job. What can a*
> *person say to a dear little widow at the*
> *mortuary who persists in asking, "Don't*
> *you want to see how natural he looks?"*
> *when "No thank you" doesn't even register?*

You may well not get any answer more potent than, "Well, gee, I don't know," which often accompanies a need to go get more ice. You may get a breezy, "Don't go to a mortuary in the first place." But even so, you must see the glimmer of hope in a solution better than the none you have now. It's a beginning.

Let's carry the mortuary question further, as an example of how you might weigh out for yourself your own future actions. (If going to the mortuary is not an issue for you, I hope you will apply the process to something else that is.) In my community, some of the advantages of going to the mortuary are that

1) hours for visiting are usually compatible with work;

2) your name on the register says for all time that you knew and cared enough to come; and

3) the mortuary gives you a chance to speak

with the family, a chance that probably won't arise at the funeral itself.

Your friends may bring up other arguments in favor of making an effort to go: what if you know there are not many friends, or what if the weather is bad and you're sure very few people will go? Is it a kindness, in your mind, to go even though you would rather visit the family at home instead?

You will almost invariably be asked to view the body. If this is difficult for you, can you comfortably decline? Or if it is expected, would it be better for you to stay away altogether?

If your heart says go, then go, feeling strengthened by your resolve and by knowing it is *your* decision. If not, you might think out a different way to make your caring evident: *I could offer to stay at my friend's home during visitation hours.* (It is a sorry fact that burglars keep an eye on obituary notices.)

You can see why my decisions, or anyone else's, cannot work by themselves as an answer to what *you* should do. An outside advisor's "shoulds" and "don'ts" wouldn't suit your comfort level, or your faith, or your community's standards. You will have to sift out your own mix, and to do that, if you're like most of your brethren in the human race, you need to talk out your ideas.

So please leave your mind open. Turn your back on the old unspoken agreement that we never talk about death. You won't arrive at hard-and-fast, for-always answers to those questions you keep asking yourself. But you *will* be more sure of your own feelings. You'll be readier to face the next shock of a death by directing your energy toward helping from your heart instead of floundering with the "mechanics" of our rituals. You'll think right past "should I . . ." and "must I . . ." to your own best ways for offering a leaning place.

I can't make your straight line, but I *can* suggest ways to give practical help after you have made your own.

Where to Begin

As a starting point, I'm convinced that you shouldn't be afraid to make any genuine offer if it seems to you like a way to help, regardless of "raised eyebrows" and regardless of what anyone else does.

How better can I reinforce that point than to recommend the telephone, an object you've already heard my reservations about. (I'm still leery of phone calls. I suppose you could say I was marked unfairly the morning after the death of my mother, by the following call: "Hello . . . this is Mrs. Mickleberry. You don't know me but I knew your mother for years. I saw in today's paper where she died. What'd she die of?")

But now I am sincere in suggesting that the phone is a helpful link. I make a point of telling my sad friends, especially if they are going to be alone, that the phone is right by my bed, that I can talk or answer their call by going to their overwhelmed selves just to *SIT,* if either will help. I add that I go back to sleep very quickly and that I won't think them a bit "weak" if they do call. In the thousand years or more, it seems, since I first found out what nights can be like after a death has swamped my own moorings, I suppose maybe two friends have called "just to talk." I think I've learned, though, that the offer does help.

The same goes for volunteering to stay over. Rarely, rarely will our friends want our physical presence. The support, even when it's welcome, may be negated by feeling the need to entertain, and knowing that facing the loss alone will still be waiting. Too, our friends vary in their capacity to accept sympathy. Ask if you can stay, if it seems a kind and gentle way to show your love. You can give assurances that you'll just be there, with your book, not expecting any attention, or even instant breakfast.

Providing Transportation

You can make yourself very useful by volunteering to take neighbors together to the services, especially when there are elderly persons in that group. If your idea seems good to the family, maybe for no better reason than the usually limited parking, then you yourself can communicate the plan and the method/time to those involved.

I carried out this idea once in a neighborhood of long-time residents and my offer was so gratefully received that I wound up enlisting two other close friends with their cars. The extraordinary amount of appreciation expressed by those who enjoyed going with someone, going into the service with someone, talking with someone made a lasting impression on me.

If out-of-town relatives or friends are coming, you could offer a run to and from the airport. You could, if this fits, arrange to take the family's car to make that run and have it washed on the way.

Bringing Umbrellas

Especially if there are out-of-town visitors, you could borrow a few umbrellas from your friends and have them on hand in case it rains the day of the funeral. You can be sure none of the out-of-towners packed an umbrella and almost as sure that of the three or four usually in the suddenly stricken home, one is at the office, one won't work, and one is very small and has a Donald Duck on it.

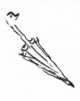

Be sure that your name is firmly attached to the borrowed umbrellas, and that *you* retrieve them afterwards. Little things mean a lot!

Warming the House

You could take your lead from my friend Grace, even if you will be attending the service. Arrange by yourself, or with a small group of good good friends, to park close to the Sanctuary, to sit in the rear, and to hurry straight to the home and be there, lights on and house warming up, when the sorrow-numbed person who will now live there alone returns from the service.

Your group could also arrange for food, as a group of my friends did for me. I fear I hadn't thought of food or of friends' calling even though I'd been through the "afterwards syndrome" enough that both should have been at the top of my mind. But I'd never done any of the planning alone before. And the gift of thoughtfulness from those friends who thought *for* me was immeasurably valuable.

Bringing Food

So let's look at food as a practical help. For some good souls, bless them, food as a way to help is an instinctive response. It must be in their genes, left over from horse-and-buggy days when families packed scads of food for the long trip to the home of a friend — some of it for themselves, but much of it to literally "put food on the table." Today, even though take-outs and drive-ins are right around every corner, I think there's a good reason that the spirit of the custom has survived. Lovingly shared food bonds friends and families, even when there are no words to express their shared loss.

Then, too, as my friend Emmy put it in one of our group's conversations on the subject, "I think it's a good idea because having food makes a start on getting a household back to normal."

So how to help best with food?

Try to coordinate with the family and with other friends offering food, just as you would any other time. Too much can be almost as discouraging to the otherwise-absorbed family as finding themselves with nothing to offer their assembled visitors. If you have to shoot in the dark, take a food-gift that is easily stored and preferably freezable.

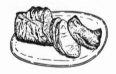

Which brings me right to my strongest suggestion: please make the containers either part of your gift or ingeniously created to self-destruct. Matching leftover containers to original concoctors gets to be hopeless as the array piles up with the help of passing time and ongoing generosity. As the recipient, you think you couldn't forget — each one of those food containers brought you such pleasure! But you're into week seven since the upheaval from Mag's death; you're on a self-imposed regime of writing thank-you notes; the regular gears of your life are gradually meshing again, only nothing quite comes smoothly yet . . . and who was it who brought the meat loaf?

You just can't picture yourself sashaying up to the front doors of various friends, asking "Will you come out to the car and pick out your Pyrex?" It sounds mighty casual for feeling as grateful as you do. And there's a good chance, too, that you'll show up at my door because I'm a good friend, but no, I didn't take any food over! Besides, the job of chauffering containers around town after a death is downright miserable.

So when you plan your food, plan to make the follow-up as simple as possible. Use an inexpensive reusable dish, or donate your container as part of the gift.

Getting Together

Think about this as a doing-gift, as we called it in Chapter 4. Aside from the fact that time is not generous in allotment of itself in the immediate aftermath of a death, your grieving friend can't be very receptive about *any*thing while struggling through the enormous number of details that need to be handled right away.

But you can plan now your gifts-of-doing for the following week . . . and for the next one after that . . . and three weeks or sixteen weeks later. Decide now how you can best reach out to your friend after the bustle of activity is over. Plan an invitation to have

-- a late breakfast;

-- a shared drive "down country" to see the autumn leaves or spring blooms;

-- a trip to the Gallery to see the Chinese exhibit;

-- a tennis match;

-- a walk with a promise of no conversation.

If you can't go-and-do, plan other ways to stay in touch with small gifts, mail, telephone.

I don't think I need to make another plea for you to *KEEP AT IT,* whatever the "it" stands for in the post-funeral reminders of your caring. You already know that a large measure of your thoughtfulness is your willingness to make it ongoing.

But please don't think you somehow demean your sincerity if you put your friend's name down on your calendar several times over the months ahead. It doesn't mean that you have to be reminded to care or sympathize; it means that you are realistic enough to know that your best intentions can get buried when the gods conspire to bring about a leak in your ceiling or a case of chicken pox in your seven-year-old. Plan now, so you'll be sure to make the time in your own busy life.

And Again, Write

Whatever else you do or don't do after a death, write. "Uh-oh," you're saying. "She's going to go off on note-writing again!" Well, you're right; I know I'm hammering away.

But if I hadn't had so much first-hand proof of how much notes help at the receiving end, I wouldn't pound, and you might not get around to doing the one thing that matters more than anything else, even a personal visit. The visit may find you talking about everything in the world but unable to say the few words that matter most to you. You can put those words in writing. And notes never interrupt, or need anyone's best efforts at putting on a sociable face, or have to be fed and coffeed and entertained.

Sometime during the first week, write a brief sympathy note. It may be a short note about the service, or a favorite quotation of yours. (My own is, *To live in the hearts of others is not to die.*) It may be just one line: *My thoughts and prayers are with you,* or: *Do know that you have all our love.*

Then get your breath and consider a second note a bit later, and then another . . . .

After Lee died, a close friend showed me a lovely way of sharing her feelings for our lost friend. Shortly after the funeral, she planted a tree in Lee's memory in a nearby city park. (If you want to make a similar gift, be sure to get permission from the Parks Department of your community. Often they will handle the selection of the tree and the planting as well, for a fee.)

In her note to me several weeks after the funeral, this friend mentioned the tree and asked if she could come by "next Wednesday at one" and join me for a walk through the park to show me where she'd planted it. Even at the time, I appreciated how gracefully she had carried out her plan. You don't have to afford an elm if you like the idea. A selection of bulbs in your own yard could make the same thought work.

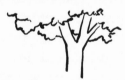

Try not to cut off the written reminders of your love and awareness after your first sympathy note. Of course, if your friend is someone you continue to see every week, you won't mail out "I'm thinking of you" messages between meetings. But if your grieving friend is far from the center of your daily whirl, remember that the lonely months after a death are, in a very real way, a long convalescence. An unexpected bouquet of flowers, or a note that says *I know it doesn't seem to get easier, but you're doing a super job,* or *This seemed a good day to send you my special love* will bring your friend the steadying assurance of knowing that his, or her, heavy heart hasn't become just "old news" to the rest of the world. Of course it hasn't, not to you, but it's easy to forget how much good it does to *SAY* it.

"Remembering" Letters

There's one more big-*BIG* way you can use the Postal Service to reach out a hand in sorrow— and you're the only one who can do it, so I hope you'll take on the job. There aren't any formal requirements, but it does take quiet time for reflection about the friend who has died, and a willingness to let your mind go back over the years as you remember having that friend as a very important part of your everyday world.

Maybe you first knew him in elementary school, maybe she was your best friend in college, maybe you worked your way up the ranks together at the accounting firm, or you met when they moved in next door and the moving van flattened your flower bed . . . some place the friendship started that leaves you now with great memories and a large lump in your chest. Let those memories count now.

This is a "remembering" letter. You write it for

the parents, wife, children, husband. And you write it for yourself, as your personal tribute. This gift is made to order for those who admit that the dash is their favorite punctuation mark — or even their only one. And if you never really bothered to get the hang of paragraphing, this writing job is for you.

You can start with something as easy to put down as

> *I think of Amy so often. I remember once . . .*

Or:
> *My brother and your Jon were the greatest friends a younger guy could ever have had. I remember the time they both . . .*

And then you'll find this letter almost writes itself as you recall the fine and funny moments, the loved qualities, special clothes, favorite expressions . . . every kind of memory that surfaces in your mind as you let it turn toward the friend you have lost.

> *I never knew anyone else who could stay wide awake through an opera and snore through James Bond.*

> *Mary taught me most of what I know about sticking to your guns —that awful car salesman —remember how she'd . . . ?*

No topic sentences, no brakes on your heart because of the structural requirements you learned in English 2A. You just write as you think, picking out brief moments, small bits and pieces, without any order of time or importance.

You can write this letter weeks or even months after a death. Sharing your memories with the family is a beautiful, one-of-a-kind gift, and a gift to yourself as well.

You may have noticed that my suggestions for what you can do to help after a death, once you have gotten over the hurdle of how you will handle the immediate demands, have a ring of familiarity from earlier chapters. I hope such familiarity is a welcome ally now, when you find yourself up against the biggest and hardest of all the troubled times you want to help your friends through. It's good to realize that your resources for helping, even now, are old friends. The starting point is a constant, whether your concern is with a broken bone or with a broken heart, or with a friend who has suffered the cruelest break of all, a loss to death.

You start from this: someone you care about is hurting, and you are unwilling to stand on the sidelines, helpless witness to that pain.

You know now, I hope, that you *can* help, that in fact there is so much you can do that you need never resort to that sad old catch-all, Well . . . if there's anything I can do . . . .

True, you can't make an illness go away. None of us can change death. But we all have the capacity to make a big difference in how our friends cope with the inevitable breakdowns of their frail human selves. We have our voices, our written words, the warmth of our presence, our offerings of time and energy, food, gifts, a listening ear . . . an open mind. Your mind teamed with your heart —it's a great combination! And great to be able to call on as you grow in ability to help your friends, after a death and for all times.

Index

H - M

P

Dates to Remember

JANUARY

NAME AND DATE   ADDRESS/TELEPHONE

FEBRUARY

ADDRESS/TELEPHONE

MARCH

APRIL

NAME AND DATE   ADDRESS/TELEPHONE

MAY

JUNE

NAME AND DATE   **ADDRESS/TELEPHONE**

NAME AND DATE	ADDRESS/TELEPHONE

AUGUST

NAME AND DATE   ADDRESS/TELEPHONE

SEPTEMBER

NAME AND DATE   ADDRESS/TELEPHONE

OCTOBER

NAME AND DATE   ADDRESS/TELEPHONE

NOVEMBER

NAME AND DATE   ADDRESS/TELEPHONE

DECEMBER